The Delphi Te
in Nursing and Health
Research

Sinead Keeney

Senior Lecturer, Institute of Nursing Research,
School of Nursing, University of Ulster, UK

Felicity Hasson

Senior Lecturer, Institute of Nursing Research,
School of Nursing, University of Ulster, UK

Hugh McKenna

Dean of Faculty of Life and Health Sciences,
University of Ulster, UK

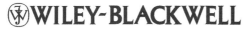

WILEY-BLACKWELL

A John Wiley & Sons, Ltd., Publication

Registered office
John Wiley & Sons Ltd, The Atrium, Southern Gate, Chichester, West Sussex, PO19 8SQ, United Kingdom

Editorial offices
9600 Garsington Road, Oxford, OX4 2DQ, United Kingdom
The Atrium, Southern Gate, Chichester, West Sussex, PO19 8SQ, UK
2121 State Avenue, Ames, Iowa 50014-8300, USA

For details of our global editorial offices, for customer services and for information about how to apply for permission to reuse the copyright material in this book please see our website at www.wiley.com/wiley-blackwell.

Library of Congress Cataloging-in-Publication Data
Keeney, Sinead.
    The Delphi technique in nursing and health research/Sinead Keeney, Felicity Hasson, Hugh McKenna.
        p. ; cm.
    Includes bibliographical references and index.
    ISBN 978-1-4051-8754-1 (pbk. : alk. paper) 1. Nursing–Research–Methodology.
2. Health–Research–Methodology.   3. Delphi method.   I. Hasson, Felicity.
II. McKenna, Hugh P., 1954-   III. Title.
    [DNLM: 1. Nursing Research–methods.   2. Delphi Technique.   3. Health Services
Research–methods.   4. Research Design. WY 20.5]
    RT81.5.K47 2011
    610.73072–dc22

                                                                            2010040520

A catalogue record for this book is available from the British Library.

Set in 9.5/12.5pt Palatino by Aptara® Inc., New Delhi, India

1   2011

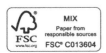

Contents

Preface

The Delphi Technique in Nursing and Health Research is written as a guide for any students and/or researchers who wish to use this methodological approach. The aim of the book is to introduce the researcher to the 'Delphi', outline its historical development and serve as a manual to facilitate the use of the technique. Issues that a Delphi researcher must consider will be presented in a straightforward fashion by discussing in detail applications to research. The reader is taken on a step-by-step journey from the research question to choosing a sample through conducting and analysing data. For example, methodology and issues related to design typologies, sampling, instrumentation, methodological rigour and methods of data analysis are discussed. Parameters for the successful application of the Delphi and its variety of uses are analysed, using examples of real empirical investigations.

The technique's key characteristics, anonymity, use of experts and controlled feedback are examined. Furthermore, the specific role of the Delphi researcher will be explored in depth. The book provides the reader with the necessary information to participate in and conduct studies using the Delphi methodology. Brief case scenarios are presented for readers' consideration. In addition, key learning points are detailed at the end of each chapter along with an extensive and current annotated bibliography.

Acknowledgements

This book is a collective creation and, as authors, we recognise the benefit from the support and labour of others.

Hugh acknowledges his wife, Tricia, his son, Gowain, and his daughter, Saoirse, whose patience and support know no bounds.

Felicity thanks her family for the support and encouragement they provided in the writing and production of this text.

Sinead thanks her husband, Declan, and her children, Niamh and Niall, for their unwavering support, belief and encouragement.

1 The Delphi Technique

Introduction

Most research studies are driven by research questions that need answering. To do so, the researcher must employ a research design. While there is little agreement among researchers as to the proper classification, Parahoo (2006) suggested that there are three types of research designs: experimental, case study and survey designs.

Experimental designs tend to be future oriented and the researcher often has to set up the conditions under which the investigation will take place. The most 'scientific' version of the experiment involving human subjects is the double-blind randomised clinical trial. It is employed widely in medicine in the testing of new drugs and is often referred to as the gold standard of research designs.

Case studies are in-depth investigations of phenomena. This type of design helps researchers gain an intimate knowledge of a person's or a group's condition, thoughts, feelings, actions both past and present, intentions and environment (Creswell, 2003).

Survey designs are by far the most common type used in health care research. This may be classified as descriptive, exploratory or comparative. The aim of a survey is to gather data from specific individuals, groups or populations for the purpose of addressing a particular issue. A more detailed overview of survey designs can be found in McKenna et al. (2006).

One type of survey that is gaining in recognition and popularity is the Delphi Technique and that is the focus of this book. This chapter will define and describe the technique, provide background as to its origins and outline the different types of Delphi surveys available to researchers. The characteristics of the Delphi will be outlined and there will be discussions on who can be categorised as experts, what constitutes a round, how feedback is handled and what is meant by anonymity and consensus. Finally, the Delphi will be compared with other consensus reaching methodologies including the nominal group technique and the consensus conference.

The Delphi Technique in Nursing and Health Research, First Edition, © S. Keeney, F. Hasson and H. McKenna   Published 2011 by Blackwell Publishing Ltd.

History of the technique

The desire for humankind to predict their future is an ongoing quest. Dating back thousands of years, oracles had a firm place in the life of Greeks and Romans. One of the most important oracles in the classical Greek world was at 'Delphi'. The Greek word *Delphois* refers to the womb indicating the Grandmother earth (Fontenrose, 1978). The name 'Delphi' is derived from the Oracle of Delphi. Delphi is an archaeological site in Greece on the south-western face of Mount Parnassus. In Greek mythology, Delphi was the location of the most important oracle in the classical Greek world, and a major site for the worship of the god Apollo. The god Apollo made himself master of Delphi, after slaying the dragon Pathos who protected the site, was also famous for his ability to foresee the future (Linstone, 1978). Legend has it that Apollo prophesies were transmitted through female intermediaries, known as *Pythia*, a name derived from the python, a source of wisdom in ancient Greece (von der Gracht, 2008). She had to be an older woman of blameless life chosen from among the peasants of the area.

In a state of trance, induced by vapours rising from a chasm in the rock, the Pythia (or priestess) would sit on a tripod over an opening in the earth and would communicate Apollo's answers to priests who would translate these back to the petitioners. People from far and wide consulted the Delphic oracle on a range of topics including important matters of public policy, to personal affairs, to the outcome of wars and the founding of colonies. Therefore, the term 'Delphi' has become synonymous with receiving good judgement on an issue.

The Delphi technique itself was developed at the beginning of the cold war to forecast the impact of technology on warfare (Custer *et al.*, 1999). In 1944, General Henry Arnold commissioned a report for the US Air Force on the future technological capabilities that might be used by the military.

Two years later, the Douglas Aircraft Company started Project RAND to study inter-continental warfare. Different approaches were tried, but the shortcomings of traditional forecasting methods, such as theoretical approaches, quantitative models or trend extrapolation, in areas where precise scientific laws have not been established yet, quickly became apparent. Similarly, exploring the use of focus groups to forecast events indicated three main problems including the influence of dominant personalities, noise and group pressure (Dalkey, 1969a).

To combat these shortcomings, the Delphi method was developed, essentially founded on the premise that individual statistical predictions were stronger than unstructured, face to face group predictions (Kaplan *et al.*, 1949). Entitled Project RAND during the 1950–1960s (1959) by Olaf Helmer, Norman Dalkey and Nicholas Rescher (Rescher, 1998) the Delphi method started to develop. Initial application of the method required experts to provide their opinion on the probability, frequency and intensity of possible enemy attacks and the number of atomic bombs needed to destroy a particular target. This process was repeated several times until a consensus emerged.

Whilst Helmer and Dalkey developed the method, Abraham Kaplan, a qualified philosopher employed by the RAND Corporation, coined the name 'Delphi'. The founders of the method, however, were critical of the name 'Delphi'. As Dalkey (1969a, p. 8) explained:

> In some ways it is unfortunate – it connotes someone oracular, something smacking a little of the occult – whereas as a matter of fact, precisely the opposite is involved; it primarily is concerned with making the best you can of a less than perfect fund of information.

Nevertheless, since the Delphi's development, there has been a broadening of the technique and it is now commonly used across a wide range of disciplines including health, nursing and medical research. The use of the Delphi technique to identify research priorities and gain consensus in many areas of health research is clearly apparent (Edwards, 2002; Sowell, 2000; Palmer & Batchelor, 2006; Byrne *et al.*, 2008).

What is the Delphi technique?

The main premise of the Delphi method is based on the assumption that group opinion is more valid than individual opinion. A novel and contemporary way of illustrating this is through the use of 'ask the audience' in the popular game show, *Who Wants to Be a Millionaire?*, where the audience effectively act as the 'expert panel', experts in general knowledge, and the contestant asks the audience for their opinion on a certain question. The audience is asked to vote on the answer using a keypad and the results displayed in a bar chart form showing where the consensus lies. Obviously, the use of the word 'expert' is used loosely here but this demonstrates the main premise of the Delphi Technique that group opinion is considered more 'valid' and 'reliable' than individual opinion.

Defining the Delphi technique

The Delphi technique has been defined as a multi-staged survey which attempts ultimately to achieve consensus on an important issue (McKenna,

1994a). Prior to this, Dalkey and Helmer (1963) asserted that the Delphi was a method used to obtain the most reliable consensus of opinion of a group of experts by a series of intensive questionnaires interspersed with controlled feedback. In essence, all definitions agree that the purpose of the technique is to achieve agreement among a group of experts on a certain issue where none previously existed.

The original advocates of the Delphi Technique, Dalkey and Helmer (1963), defined the Delphi technique as 'a method used to obtain the most reliable consensus of opinion of a group of experts by a series of intensive questionnaires interspersed with controlled feedback' (p. 458). With increasing usage, broader definitions have been put forward. For instance, Reid (1998) believed that Delphi is a method for the systematic collection and aggregation of informed judgement from a group of experts on specific questions and issues.

Lynn *et al.* (1998) defined the Delphi technique as an iterative process designed to combine expert opinion into group consensus. Most definitions attempt to encompass or highlight the ever-adapting Delphi process in one sentence, which has resulted in broad and varying interpretations of the technique. Regardless of definition, as alluded to above the purpose of the technique is to achieve consensus among a group of experts on a certain issue where no agreement previously existed.

There are many differing forms of Delphi now in existence, such as the 'modified Delphi' (Rauch, 1979; McKenna, 1994a), the 'policy Delphi' (Crisp *et al.*, 1997), and the 'real-time Delphi' (Beretta, 1996). Few researchers now use a uniform method of the Delphi technique, and this has been heavily criticised since the emergence of modifications of the technique poses a threat to the credibility of the Delphi technique and the validity and reliability of the research findings (Sackman, 1975).

The Delphi process

Original Delphi

In its original form, the Delphi process consists of two or more rounds of questionnaires administrated by post to an expert panel. The first questionnaire asks the expert panel for their opinions on a certain issue or topic in an open-ended manner. These responses are then analysed by the researchers and sent back to the expert panel in the form of statements or questions. The expert panel rate or rank the statements or questions within the second questionnaire according to their expert opinion on the subject. Rounds continue until a consensus is reached on some or all of the items as required. Today, this is known as the Classical Delphi.

Idea generation

This original approach sets the foundation for an idea-generation strategy to uncover the issues pertaining to the topic under study. To do this, the respondents, referred to as panellists or experts, are asked to put forward as many relevant issues as possible in Round 1. Once analysed, these responses act as a springboard for the rest of the Delphi process. Feedback from Round 1 is provided in the form of a second questionnaire and opinion is asked on the issues raised. Normally, in subsequent rounds each panel member is provided with their own responses as well as those of the other panellists or experts and he or she is asked to reconsider and (if they wish) change it in the light of other panellists' responses. This continues for subsequent rounds until consensus is obtained. This process is best described as multi-stage where each stage builds on the results of the previous one (Sumsion, 1998).

Priority setting versus consensus

The Delphi technique is used for two main purposes within nursing and health research. Firstly, it is commonly used to set priorities, for example the identification of nursing research priorities. Nurses, academics and researchers could form an expert panel to identify research priorities for the nursing profession at present. There are a large number of studies that have been undertaken in this area across the world (e.g. French *et al.*, 2002; Griffen-Sobel & Suozzo, 2002; McIlfatrick & Keeney, 2003; Cohen *et al.*, 2004; Annells *et al.*, 2005; Back-Pettersson *et al.*, 2008; Grundy & Ghazi, 2009). This type of priority setting exercise can be useful for the profession or experts involved or for funders to prioritise what areas of research should be funded in the short, medium and long term.

The second main use of the Delphi technique is to gain consensus. This can be on any set of issues or ideas. The expert panel are asked to rank or rate items either generated by themselves within Round 1 of the Delphi, as in the Classical Delphi, or in a modified Delphi through the literature or the use of focus groups or interviews. A consensus level is set (e.g. 70%) and once the pre-determined percentage of the expert panel has come to agreement on the importance or position of the statement, it is said to have reached consensus. Consensus studies have been widely utilised in nursing and health research to date (e.g. Butterworth & Bishop, 1995; Beech, 1997; Graham *et al.*, 2003; Beattie *et al.*, 2004; Cornick, 2006; Ferguson *et al.*, 2008; Jorm *et al.*, 2008).

Non-consensus Delphi

While it may not appear immediately relevant to nursing or health research, it is important to point out that not all Delphi's aim to reach consensus. Traditionally, the method has aimed at gaining consensus but other Delphi's, such as the Policy Delphi, aim to support decisions by structuring and discussing the diverse views of the 'preferred future' (Turoff, 2006). The Argument Delphi, a derivative of the Policy Delphi (Kuusi, 1999), focuses on ongoing discussion and seeking relevant arguments rather than focusing on the output. The 'Disaggregative Policy Delphi' (Tapio, 2002) uses cluster analysis as a systematic tool to construct various scenarios of the future in the latest Delphi round.

Types of Deplhi

How has the Delphi evolved?

Since its inception the Delphi technique has evolved into a number of modifications (see Table 1.1). There are hundreds and possibly thousands of studies in the literature reporting on studies using these different manifestations, and this is tribute to the flexibility of the method.

The reason for these adaptations is based on the fact that there are no formal, universally agreed guidelines on the use of the Delphi. Its original form, known as the *classical Delphi*, involves the presentation of a questionnaire to a panel of 'informed individuals' in a specific field of application, in order to seek their opinion or judgement on a particular issue. After they respond, the data are summarised and a new questionnaire is designed based solely on the results obtained from the first round. This second instrument is returned to each subject and they are asked (in the light of the first round's results), to reconsider their initial opinion and to once again return their responses to the researcher. Repeat rounds of this process may be carried out until consensus of opinion, or a point of diminishing returns, has been reached. This illustrates the Delphi technique is a multi-stage approach with each stage building on the results of the previous one. Hitch and Murgatroyd (1983) saw it resembling a highly controlled meeting of experts, facilitated by a chairperson who is adept at summing up the feelings of the meeting by reflecting the participants' own views back to them in such a way that they can proceed further – the only difference is that the individual responses of the members are unknown to one another. A *classical Delphi* format was employed by McIlfatrick and Keeney (2003) with 112 nurses attending a cancer nursing research conference in Northern Ireland. The aim of this survey was for those attending to identify priorities for cancer research.

Nevertheless, it is widely used in a great variety of forms (Mead, 1991; Butterworth & Bishop, 1995; Green *et al.*, 1999) without adequate consideration of the consequences. For further reading of the numerous variations of formats of the Delphi, see Chien *et al.* (1984).

Table 1.1   Types of Delphi's and main characteristics

Classical Delphi	Uses an open first round to facilitate idea generation to elicit opinion and gain consensus
	Uses three or more postal rounds
	Can be administered by email
Modified Delphi	Modification usually takes the form of replacing the first postal round with face-to-face interviews or focus group
	May use fewer than three postal or email rounds
Decision Delphi	Same process usually adopted as a classical Delphi
	Focuses on making decisions rather than coming to consensus
Policy Delphi	Uses the opinions of experts to come to consensus and agree future policy on a given topic
Real Time Delphi	Similar process to classical Delphi except that experts may be in the same room
	Consensus reached in real time rather than by post
	Sometimes referred to as a consensus conference
e-Delphi	Similar process to the classical Delphi but administered by email or online web survey
Technological Delphi	Similar to the real time Delphi but using technology, such as hand held keypads allowing experts to respond to questions immediately while the technology works out the mean/median and allows instant feedback allowing experts the chance to re-vote moving towards consensus in the light of group opinion
Online Delphi	Same process at classical Delphi but questionnaires are completed and submitted online
Argument Delphi	Focused on the production of relevant factual arguments
	Derivative of the Policy Delphi
	Non-consensus Delphi
Disaggregative Delphi	Goal of consensus not adopted
	Conducts various scenarios of the future for discussion
	Uses cluster analysis

Source: Keeney (2009).

Sampling and the use of experts

Defining 'expert'

The fact that the Delphi does not always use a random sample which is representative of the target population is a point that must be given consideration by researchers; rather, it employs 'experts'. This means that each respondent is an expert in the area in which the researcher is interested. An expert has been defined as a group of 'informed individuals' (McKenna, 1994a) and as 'specialists' in their field (Goodman, 1987) or someone who has knowledge about a specific subject (Davidson *et al.*, 1997; Lemmer, 1998; Green *et al.*, 1999). For example, a study investigating the role of the health visitor may include health visitors who are knowledgeable about the subject under consideration (Lemmer, 1998).

Employing an expert panel

The identification of experts has been a major point of debate in the use of the 'Delphi'. Since deciding on the makeup of the expert panel is the first stage in the Delphi process, the formation of this panel is regarded as the 'lynchpin of the method' (Green *et al.*, 1999, p. 200). However, it is also the selection of the expert sample that raises methodological concerns. Sackman (1975) criticised the use of experts as did Linstone and Turoff (1975) and McKenna (1994a). The claim of the 'Delphi' to represent valid expert opinion has been criticised as scientifically untenable and overstated (Strauss & Zeigler, 1975a). It is not surprising that Linstone (Linstone, 1975; Linstone & Turoff 1975) refers to the pitfall of 'illusory expertise' (p. 566) and Goodman (1987) warned about the 'potentially misleading title of expert' (p. 732).

Simply because individuals have knowledge of a particular topic does not necessarily mean that they are experts. In fact, those who are willing to engage in discussion are more likely to be affected directly by the outcome of the process and are also more likely to become and stay involved in the Delphi. Hence, the commitment of participants is related to their interest and involvement with the question or issue being addressed. However, respondents must be relatively impartial so that the information obtained reflects current knowledge or perceptions (Goodman, 1987). This balance is difficult to achieve and justify to the consumers of the finished research. There is also little agreement about the size of the expert panel, the relationship of the panel to the larger population of experts and the sampling method used to select such experts (Williams & Webb, 1994a, 1994b).

Size of the expert panel

Sample size and heterogeneity depends upon the purpose of the project, design selected and time frame for data collection (Goodman, 1987; McKenna, 1994a; Green *et al.*, 1999). For the conventional Delphi, a heterogeneous sample is used to ensure that the entire spectrum of opinion is determined (Moore, 1987). Sampling different groups of experts, such as nurse educators and nurse students (Sullivan & Brye, 1983), may ensure heterogeneity.

It is becoming increasingly frequent for Delphi researchers to employ clear inclusion criteria to create boundaries around their expert panel (Keeney *et al.*, 2001, 2006). The inclusion criteria can include, for example specific qualifications, number of publications in the area of expertise, geographical location or years experience in a particular area.

Valid opinion

One of the most important things that any researcher using the Delphi technique must remember is that this method elicits valid opinion from experts in the area. An opinion is a belief that may or may not be backed up with evidence but which cannot be proved with any evidence that may exist. The Delphi technique does not produce any right or wrong answers or any definitive answers; instead, it produces valid expert opinion.

It is assumed that the Delphi technique 'works' due to the feedback given to the expert panel and the quasi-anonymity afforded to the panel (Rowe *et al.*, 2005). This feedback allows the panel to consider the group response and their own response in the light of this. It is at this point that an expert panel member may 'change' or modify their opinion, having considered the group opinion, and the panel may move towards consensus.

Anonymity

Anonymity provides an equal chance for each panel member to present and react to ideas unbiased by the identities of other participants (Goodman, 1987). Reactions are given independently; so each opinion carries the same weight and is given equal importance in the analysis. In this way, subject bias is eliminated, as the respondents are not known to each other (Goodman, 1987; Jeffery *et al.*, 1995). This promise of anonymity facilitates respondents to be open and truthful about their views on certain issues, which in turn provides insightful data for the researcher. Furthermore, Couper (1984) suggested that this provides each participant with an opportunity to express an opinion to others without feeling pressured psychologically by the more influential panel members. It is unclear at present whether respondents in a Delphi process change their opinions on the basis of new information or, despite the protection of anonymity, feel pressurised to conform to the group's view. Complete anonymity may lead to a lack of accountability for the views expressed, thus encouraging ill-considered judgements (Goodman, 1987).

Quasi-anonymity

Complete anonymity cannot be guaranteed when using the Delphi technique; a fact that many studies do not address. Firstly, the researcher knows the panel members and their responses; this in itself threatens true anonymity. Secondly, it is often the case that panel members know each other, but they cannot attribute responses to any one member. It is like being in an elite 'expert' club where the membership is known but they do not meet face to face to discuss the issues. In fact, knowing that you are a member of an exclusive club may help motivate panellists to participate. McKenna (1994a) used the term 'quasi-anonymity' when the respondents may be known to one another, but their judgements and opinions remain strictly anonymous. Anonymity has recently been questioned by other Delphi users, such as Sumsion (1998), who recommended that a 70% response rate is obtained for each round: to achieve this respondents and non-respondents must be known. The influence of anonymity upon findings has not to the authors' knowledge been reported in the Delphi literature.

Group dynamics

Group dynamics is a general term used to describe group processes. A group is considered to be two or more individuals who are connected to each other by some form of relationship. Members of groups interact and influence one another and due to this groups develop a number of dynamic processes that separates them from a random collection of individuals. Such processes could include roles, relationships, development and influence.

The group dynamics within a Delphi study exist with the expert panel. They have several things in common; they are a member of the panel and have knowledge and insight into the same area of expertise. They may even work together in a geographical tight Delphi. Even if they are world experts in a narrow field, they may be well known to each other. These factors can produce influence by one panel member over another in later rounds of the technique when group feedback is provided to the expert panel. This influence can result in individuals changing their opinion to come into line with the group and, hence, converge on consensus on identified issues.

Delphi rounds

As discussed above, the Delphi technique employs a number of rounds in which questionnaires are sent out and are used until consensus is reached (Beretta, 1996; Green *et al.*, 1999). In each round, a summary of the results of the previous round is included and evaluated by the panel members. McKenna (1994a) implies that this process facilitates the 'systematic emergence of a concurrence of judgement/opinion' (p. 1222). The number of rounds depends upon the time available and whether the experimenter commenced the Delphi sequence with one broad question or with a list of questions or events. The process raises the question of how many rounds it takes to reach consensus. The classical original Delphi used four rounds (Young & Hogben, 1978). However, this has been modified by many to suit individual research aims and, in some cases, it has been shortened to two or three rounds (Proctor & Hunt, 1994; Beech, 1997; Green *et al.*, 1999). It is difficult to retain a high response rate within a 'Delphi' that has many rounds. The topic needs to be of great interest to the panel members or they have to be rewarded in other ways.

Round 1

Round 1 of the classical Delphi starts with an open-ended set of questions, thus allowing panel members freedom in their responses. The number of items generated can be extremely large, especially if the researcher opts for an inclusive approach. Supporting this Proctor and Hunt (1994) stated that the Delphi process can produce 'large and unwieldy amounts of information particularly if the researcher adopts a qualitative stance towards the data and is reluctant to collapse categories' (p. 1004). Unfortunately, this tendency to include all the panel members' Round 1 views can create second round questionnaires of over 25 pages. Being all inclusive can put panel members off participating and can become very difficult to sustain (Green *et al.*, 1999). A further critique concerns the view that if questions are not well phrased and definitive, the reliability and validity of data may be threatened. Reliability and validity of the Delphi are discussed in detail in Chapter 7.

Traditionally, Round 1 is used to generate ideas and the panel members are asked for their responses to or comments about an issue. There is now some support for revising the approach and providing pre-existing information for ranking or response. However, it must be recognised that this approach could bias the responses or limit the available options. Nonetheless, a clear advantage to commencing the process in this way is that it could be more efficient in a technique that has the potential to be very time consuming (Duffield, 1993; Jenkins & Smith, 1994).

Subsequent rounds

Rounds 2–4 often take the form of structured questionnaires incorporating feedback to each panel member. These rounds are analysed and recirculated, and it has been shown that this process encourages panel members to become more involved and motivated to participate (Walker & Selfe, 1996). In this way, the Delphi allows efficient and rapid collection of expert opinions, while the feedback is controlled (Buck *et al.*, 1993).

The ability of the Delphi to involve and motivate panel members means that they can be involved actively in the development of the instrument: this leads to perceptions of ownership and acceptance of the findings (McKenna, 1994a). The active involvement of staff in the identification of their own development needs is crucial for the success of any development program (Shepard, 1995). This can be viewed as an incentive and major advantage in using this technique.

The Delphi often collects qualitative and quantitative data yet little guidance exists in relation to the balance of data collected and how to manage the data generated (Green *et al.*, 1999). The lack of guidance leads to a variety of approaches and can result in different Delphi studies interpreting and reporting in different ways: this could affect the integrity of the method.

The Delphi technique might encounter problems due to a decline in response rate because, in order to achieve consensus, it is important that those panel members who have agreed to participate stay involved until the process is completed (Buck *et al.*, 1993). However, poor response rates are a characteristic of the final round of the Delphi. This has been a perennial criticism and could be an explanation as to why many researchers are now stopping at two or three rounds rather than the originally recommended four rounds. McKenna (1994a), however, found that using face-to-face interviews in the first round increases the return rates of postal questionnaires in the second.

Response rates

Enhancing response rate

In general, questionnaire research is notorious for its low response rates. Researchers often have to send out two or three reminder letters to non-responders. With anything up to four rounds of questionnaires, the Delphi asks much more of respondents than a simple survey and the potential for low response rates increases dramatically.

To enhance responses in Delphi rounds it is critical that participants realise and feel that they are partners in the study and are interested in the topic. The researcher should take every opportunity to remind participants that each round is constructed entirely on their responses to previous rounds encouraging ownership and active participation. This attempt to encourage participants to psychologically 'sign up to' a study is common in longitudinal cohort studies where researchers send regular updating newsletters to participants as well as birthday or Christmas cards. However, there could be ethical considerations with this approach as participants may feel 'forced' to continue even though they may wish to withdraw (Beretta, 1996).

McKenna (1994b) suggested that the 'personal touch' could help enhance return rates. Using face-to-face interviews as his first round, he achieved a 100% response rate, which is very rare in a Delphi study. Such a relationship is necessary to increase the likelihood of ongoing commitment from the participant. It starts at initial contact where the researcher gains informed consent and explains either in writing or verbally the nature of the research, what the participant's role is and what is required of them. Another currently emerging trend with the Delphi is a recruiting round as a preliminary round to the first 'proper' Delphi round (Hung et al., 2008). Recruiting letters should include an explanation of the study, anticipated number of rounds, outline of time commitment and a consent form or confirmation of acceptance to take part in the study. The idea behind this is to get the expert panel to sign up or even 'consent' to take part in the study before it begins. There is no evidence as yet as to whether this enhances the response rate.

The follow-up of non-respondents within a classical or modified Delphi approach is essential. Researchers' choose to do this in different ways including sending follow-up postcards or letters, a further copy of the questionnaire, or a follow-up phone call or email (McIlfatrick & Keeney, 2003; McKenna & Keeney, 2004). Prompt and appropriate feedback can also facilitate a high response rate as it keeps the members of the expert panel interested. Interest will be lost if weeks and months pass before feedback is received on the previous round.

Consensus

It is of utmost important to remember that achieving consensus on a certain issue does not mean that the correct answer has been found. It means that consensus has been reached among a panel of participants. The Delphi has been criticised as a method which forces consensus and does not allow participants to discuss issues. This means that no opportunity arises for respondents to elaborate on their views (Goodman, 1987, Walker & Selfe, 1996). However, there are other research approaches, such as focus groups that cater for discussion and elaboration. In a face-to-face discussion, there is always the disadvantage that strong-minded people or those who are more persuasive will dictate the direction of the discussion. One advantage of the Delphi is that this is avoided.

This method is not a replacement for rigorous scientific reviews of published reports or for original research. There is a danger that the 'Delphi' can lead the observer to place greater reliance on their results than might otherwise be warranted. However, as long as this is kept in mind and addressed, consensus can be gained and the Delphi can be used as a useful, integral consensus technique.

Does consensus exist in expert panels?

Expert panels are increasingly being used to determine whether or not consensus exists about many issues, for example criteria for good practice (Scott & Black, 1991). Scott and Black (1991) explored whether or not consensus exists in expert panels by establishing two expert panels to assess the appropriate indicators for cholecystectomy. Results showed that when extreme views (outliers) were eliminated agreement was fairly easy to achieve. The authors concluded that given that the overall aim of expert panels is to identify broad areas of agreement, that it would seem reasonable to disregard extreme opinions.

Concept of consensus

Consensus can have many different connotations depending on its reference. However, the concept of 'consensus' could also be termed as 'collective agreement'. It usually involves collaboration rather than compromise. Rather than opinion being adopted by a plurality, stakeholders are brought together, often with facilitation until a convergence of opinion is reached. It is important to keep in mind that a high degree of variation is possible among individuals even within consensual groups, and this can affect outcomes if action is to be taken on agreed issues.

In relation to the Delphi technique, these principles apply to the process of using the technique to gain consensus on an issue or a set of issues. Experts are brought together and the process is 'facilitated' by the researcher through the use of questionnaire rounds. Some Delphi studies have defined the concept of consensus as 'a condition of homogeneity or consistency of opinion among the panellists' (Graham *et al.*, 2003, pp. 1152–1153).

Increasing popularity in nursing and health research

The Delphi has been growing in popularity over recent years within health care research. This growth is centred on the fact that, like a questionnaire, it allows the inclusion of a large number of individuals across diverse geographic locations. However, unlike questionnaires, the Delphi aims to gain consensus of opinion, judgement or choice. The four key characteristics which are the necessary defining attributes of a Delphi technique include anonymity of response among participants, thus avoiding group dominance; iteration which allows participants to change their opinions in subsequent rounds, controlled feedback showing the distribution of the group's response and statistical group response which expresses judgement using summary measures of the full group response (Rowe & Wright, 1999). Each of these issues will be discussed in more detail in the following chapters.

A perusal of modern health care literature or a key word search in an online database uncovers a wealth of studies where the Delphi technique was employed (Green *et al.*, 1999; Alahlafi & Burge, 2005; Avery *et al.*, 2005; Mackellar *et al.*, 2007). The Delphi is often used to identify guidelines or set priorities. Bond and Bond (1982) used the technique to establish clinical nursing research priorities as did many others (Lindeman, 1975; Daniels & Ascough, 1999; Soanes *et al.*, 2000; Cohen *et al.*, 2004; Annells *et al.*, 2005). Nurse researchers were one of the first to identify the strengths of the Delphi and the number of published papers in the nursing literature is testament to that (Love, 1997; Lemmer, 1998; Moreno-Casbas *et al.*, 2001; Peters *et al.*, 2001; Sharkey & Sharples, 2001; O'Brien *et al.*, 2002; Hermann *et al.*, 2006).

Comparison of the Delphi with other consensus methods

Consensus building, also sometimes known as collaborative problem-solving or collaboration (Burgess & Spangler, 2003), is a process used to generate ideas, understand problems and to settle complex issues. Apart from the Delphi technique there are two other research approaches to achieving consensus. These include the nominal group technique (Carney *et al.*, 1996) and the consensus conference (Jones & Hunter, 1995).

Nominal group technique

The Nominal Group Technique (NGT) brings together participants for a discussion using a highly structured group approach, led by a moderator. It consists of two rounds in which panellists rate, discuss and then re-rate a series of items or issues (Jones & Hunter, 1995). The process begins with a question being posed to the group. Individually and silently, participants write their answers or ideas. These are then shared in 'round robin' fashion. This process can be repeated a number of times, with the aim of reaching a higher level of consensus. This method encourages contributions from everyone by allowing equal participation among group members (Gibson, 2001). Within the NGT, ideas are generated in a short period of time and participants can see at first hand the process of reaching consensus. According to Moore (1987), NGT is a useful method for idea generation in group discussions.

Scott and Deadrick (1982) referred to NGT as a special purpose group process appropriate for identifying elements of a problem situation, identifying elements of a solution programme and establishing priorities. According to Carney *et al.* (1996), it has a highly structured format and provides an opportunity to achieve a substantial amount of work in a relatively short space of time.

Consensus conference

Consensus conferences are organised when agreement has to be reached on a matter of importance. This could be a policy issue or an attempt to identify research priorities for a discipline. The means of doing this is to invite a purposive sample of individuals or groups to a conference venue and focus the presentations on the importance of the issue at hand and why the achievement of consensus is important. These presentations are normally followed by group work where the pros and cons of the issue at hand are discussed. The conference usually closes with a plenary session where delegates can vote or show their preference, judgement or decision on the issues.

Consensus conferences are often problematic for a number of reasons. They can be expensive to organise, selecting the correct type and number of delegates is difficult, and strong-willed individuals or groups can dictate the direction of the discussion. These limitations are offset by the importance of face-to-face discussion and the fact that everyone present is exposed to the same presentations and can better understand the context surrounding the issue requiring consensus.

Key learning points

- The Delphi method was developed originally at the beginning of the cold war to forecast the impact of technology on warfare.
- The main premise of the Delphi method is based on the assumption that group opinion is more valid than individual opinion.
- The Delphi technique is an approach used to gain consensus on a certain issue or set of issues.
- Since its inception the Delphi technique has evolved into a number of modifications.
- It does not use a random sample that is representative of the target population; rather, it employs a panel of 'experts'.
- The Delphi technique consists of a number of rounds which can be employed in different ways.
- The number of rounds depends upon how easily consensus is reached on a topic, the time available and the type of Delphi.
- The Delphi technique is not a replacement for rigorous scientific reviews of published reports or original research.
- Consensus reached using the Delphi technique does not mean that the correct answer has been found but rather that the experts have come to an agreement on the issue or issues under exploration.

Recommended further reading

Hasson, F., Keeney, S. & McKenna, H. (2000) Research guidelines for the Delphi survey technique. *Journal of Advanced Nursing* 32(4), 1008–1015.

Keeney, S., Hasson, F. & McKenna, H.P. (2001) A critical review of the Delphi technique as a research methodology for nursing. *International Journal of Nursing Studies* 38, 195–200.

Keeney, S., Hasson, F. & McKenna, H.P. (2006) Consulting the oracle: ten lessons from using the Delphi technique in nursing research. *Journal of Advanced Nursing* 53(2), 205–212.

McKenna, H.P. (1994) The Delphi technique: a worthwhile approach for nursing? *Journal of Advanced Nursing* 19, 1221–1225.

2 Debates, Criticisms and Limitations of the Delphi

Introduction

This chapter will review the key criticisms of the Delphi technique and will begin by introducing the debate on the technique's ontological position and epistemology followed by a discussion of the pitfalls to avoid. Numerous authors have reported upon the controversy surrounding this technique, and they will be outlined in this chapter. The key advantages for choosing this method are also discussed.

The qualitative-quantitative debate – which paradigm does the Delphi belong to?

Research paradigm, such as positivism, post-positivism, critical theory and constructivism, are a set (or system) of beliefs that guide how to conduct the study. In any research, it is important to identify the paradigm within which your methodology belongs; indeed, Vazquez-Ramos *et al.* (2009) claims that 'how the researcher designs and implements the Delphi method is not as important as the philosophic assumptions underlying its usage' (p. 112). However, the identification and discussion of the Delphi method epistemological stance is an aspect often neglected. The prime reason is that a classic and modified Delphi can incorporate qualitative and quantitative approaches. Therefore, it does not follow an accepted scientific procedure (Sackman, 1975) or, indeed, lend itself to the traditional scientific approach (Mullen, 2000; Powell, 2003).

Nevertheless, attempts in the literature have prescribed a positivist paradigm, which enforces the merits of the scientific inquiry (Day & Bobeva, 2005). This approach assumes that the researcher is objective and the application of single statistical measures to grade consensus. Such a case could be attributed to the Delphi as part of the data is

The Delphi Technique in Nursing and Health Research, First Edition, © S. Keeney, F. Hasson and H. McKenna   Published 2011 by Blackwell Publishing Ltd.

collected through a quantitative approach. Furthermore, Blackburn (1999) and Monti and Tingen (1999) explained that as the Delphi requires experts to agree on a single reality, the reductionist approach to the 'identification of the phenomenon under study could also be understood as adhering to positivist principles' (Hanafin, 2004, p. 7).

Other authors, however, position the Delphi technique within an interpretative paradigm, particularly social constructivism (Turoff, 1975; Rauch, 1979; Stewart, 2001; Hanafin, 2004; Engles & Kennedy, 2007; Amos & Pearse, 2008), viewing it as subjective and qualitative in nature (Fitzsimmons & Fitzsimmons, 2001). Engles and Kennedy (2007) suggest this paradigm is particularly suited to the policy Delphi (Turoff, 1975) and decision Delphi (Rauch, 1979) as both designs aim to explore divergence of views, and it aims to identify all possibilities to support later decision-making. If you accept that a Delphi study's findings are based on the constructed reality of panel members, this does not fit into reliability and validity criteria, as defined within the traditional positivist paradigm. Hanafin (2004) justifies the selection of social constructivism believing that a Delphi 'is a process of individual feedback about group opinion with opportunities for respondents to change their position primarily on the basis of that feedback, provides a close fit' (p. 8) with this paradigms assumptions. Miller and Crabtree (1992) referred to this as the constructivist inquirer within which the researcher performs 'an ongoing iterative dance of discovery and interpretation' (p. 11). The final aim is 'to distill a consensus construction that is more informed and sophisticated than any of the predecessor constructions' (Guba & Lincoln, 1998, p. 207).

Within the constructionist paradigm some view the Delphi's underpinning within the Lockean inquiry system (Churchman, 1973; Reid, 1988; Linstone, 1999) as it validates truth through human experience (Malmsjö, 2006; Engles & Kennedy, 2007). Others conceptualise a Delphi method's research questions within the Singerian inquiry system (Mitroff & Turoff, 1975; Scheele, 1975) as it assumes that 'truth is pragmatic' (Strauss & Zeigler, 1975b, p. 194) and is directly linked to the context-dependent nature of the participants' knowledge (Guba & Lincoln, 1989; Crotty, 1998).

Alternatively, Critcher and Gladstone (1998) suggested that as the Delphi derives quantitative data estimated through qualitative approaches (Bowles, 1999); it resulted in a hybrid epistemological status. Indeed, Blass (2003) claims that attempts to ground the methodology in one single paradigm is unproductive.

Over 50 years ago, Helmer and Rescher (1959) produced their seminal paper *The Epistemology of the Inexact Sciences*, which claimed that the fields have not yet developed for the Delphi approach to the point of having scientific laws or the testimony of experts to be permissible. The debate continues in the Delphi literature with no real agreement in sight.

Criticisms of the Delphi technique

The majority of early literature on the Delphi was written by its proponents and then, in 1963 Olaf Helmer, and in 1975 Harold Sackman, supported by RAND Corporation, both discussed the merits of the technique, highlighting concerns about its scientific value. Since then, the Delphi has been subject to considerable criticisms, which relate to five main areas:

1. Lack of universal guidelines
2. Size of expert panel
3. Implications of lack on anonymity
4. Expert 'opinion'
5. Level of consensus

Each of these will be discussed briefly.

Lack of universal guidelines

One key disadvantage which overarches all difficulties with the technique is the lack of scientific or professional guidelines upon which a Delphi is based. Sackman (1975) heavily criticised the approach for failing to meet virtually every major area of professional standards relating to design administration, application and validation, leading Linstone and Turoff (1975) to assert that the Delphi method is more of an art than a science.

As Turoff (1970) reported with no established rules to guide Delphi studies, the widespread use of the technique has led to numerous variations in format and implementation, which in turn has resulted in a difficulty in constructing a single definition of the approach (Linstone & Turoff, 1975; van Dijk, 1990). In a review of Delphi studies Mullen (2003) identified 23 labels being used to describe Delphi's (see Table 2.1) to which the term 'e-Delphi' should also be included. She also identified 20 variations on the way authors referred to the study including Delphi technique, survey, investigation, method and panel technique. Such variances can enhance confusion about the technique.

Although some general rules do exist which may instil confidence, such as the need to give feedback or to have at least two rounds (Day & Bobeva,

Table 2.1   Delphi labels

Delphi	Delphi conference	Goals	Fuzzy	Quantitative	Reactive
Classical	Policy	Ranking	Numerical	Variant	Modified
Conventional	Decision	Expert	Analytical	Max-min	Normative
Real-time	Historical	Delphi forecast	Exploratory	Laboratory	e-Delphi

Source: Adapted from Mullen (2003, pp. 38–39).

2005; Briedenhann & Butts, 2006; Kaynak & Marandu, 2006), these are often open to interpretation. For example a defining characteristic of the Delphi is the establishment of consensus through the feedback of panel members' individual responses and those of other panellists. It is assumed that this process allows panel members to see areas of agreement and disagreement, the opportunity to re-consider their response and to develop a complete understanding of the issue. Feedback can influence responses, therefore, the procedures need to be carefully considered. However, the format of feedback varies from a single number (Jolson & Rossow, 1971), to complete distributions (Sahal & Yee, 1975) to members comments (Clayton, 1997).

In addition, whilst two rounds are believed to be necessary to gain consensus examples of single round Delphi studies do exist. For example, Binkley *et al.* (1993) implemented a single round to gauge the level of agreement on diagnostic classification for patients with low back pain. Experts in Round 1 were presented with diagnostic categories selected from the literature and were asked to grade each classification on the appropriateness for treating the condition. In addition, 30 experts were asked to record any diagnostic groupings not included. Results from Round 2 were used to establish the level of consensus. Later Klessig *et al.* (2000) employed a single round to gain consensus on the measurement of quality in medical residency education. Round 1 included 44 items based on research evaluating such training, from which panellists were asked to rank the most important to least important. Rank outcomes determined consensus with no further rounds or additional research undertaken. Clearly, however employing more than two rounds in a Delphi is dependent upon the arrival of consensus or the point at which convergence of opinion occurs (Boyce *et al.*, 1993; Cleary, 2001).

Nevertheless, while the methods 'greyness' may be viewed by some as a key benefit, allowing flexibility in its application, this has serious repercussions for the technique's scientific respectability. Moreover, the lack of agreed guidance raises dilemmas for researchers in the field, leading some to document the problems encountered (Green *et al.*, 1999; Keeney *et al.*, 2006). While a number of authors (Jillson, 1975a; Lang, 1994; Eggers & Jones, 1998; Hasson *et al.*, 2000; Keeney *et al.*, 2006; Skulmoski *et al.*, 2007) have attempted to provide recommendations for the improvement and application of the Delphi, these are by no means universally accepted or complete.

Size of expert panel

There is no direction on the number of people required to constitute a representative sample, or the relationship to the larger sample. As a consequence the size of Delphi panels vary considerably, from under 15 (Turoff, 1970; Delbecq *et al.*, 1975; Malone *et al.*, 2005; Strasser *et al.*,

2005) to 15–100 (Rowe & Wright, 1999; Miller, 2001; Doughty, 2009), to hundreds (Cyphert & Gant, 1971; Okamoto, 1999; Kelly & Porock, 2005; Meadows *et al.*, 2005; Back-Pettersson *et al.*, 2008) and thousands of participants (Barnette *et al.*, 1978; Farrell & Scherer, 1983; NISTEP, 1997; Aichholzer, 2001; Drennan *et al.*, 2007; Jung-Erceg *et al.*, 2007; Grundy & Ghazi, 2009). A number of authors suggested a panel size should be between 8 and 12 experts (Cavalli-Sforza & Ortolano, 1984; Richey *et al.*, 1985; Novakowski & Wellar, 2008), Linstone and Turoff (1975) and Jones and Twiss (1978) recommended 10–50 participants whereas Wild and Torgersen (2000a) suggested a panel size of 300–500 provides representative information, while Parente and Anderson-Parente (1987) advocate a minimum of 10 with no upper limit.

In most research, a general rule of thumb is the more participants the better, in a Delphi study, for example Cochran (1983) professed that large panel size can enhance reliability and reduce error. However, as Murphy *et al.* (1998) stated: 'There is very little actual empirical evidence on the effect of the number of participants on the reliability or validity of consensus processes' (p. 37). Others (Delbecq *et al.*, 1975; Brooks, 1979; Fink *et al.*, 1984; Clayton, 1997) warned that increasing the group size beyond 30 has seldom been found to improve results, as large panels can be difficult to manage and result in high attrition rates (De Villiers *et al.*, 2005). Alternatively, concerns have been expressed about bias and generalisability resulting from small sample panels. For example, Synnott and McKie (1997) reported that 37 experts were too small a sample to generate a definite conclusion.

Turoff (2006) suggested that instead of asking how many experts there should be, the first question should be how many varieties of experts are needed to ensure all the relevant perspectives are included. Answering this he believed will guide the size of the panel required. Yet this raises further questions regarding the homogenous or heterogeneous composition of the expert panel. Typically, the sample size for homogeneous samples may be small (Duncan *et al.*, 2004), which Ziglio (1996) and Akins *et al.* (2005) both believed can produce sound results. Diverse, heterogeneous panels may require larger samples to ensure validity of results (Baker *et al.*, 2006).

Although the use of heterogeneity panels are advocated (Mead & Moseley, 2001; Mullen, 2003; Powell, 2003), the difficulties of adopting this approach are rarely addressed (Baker *et al.*, 2006). Essentially, without guidance, the decision on sample size is empirical and pragmatic (Thangaratinam & Redman, 2005) based on the aim of the study, resources available and design selected.

Implications of lack of anonymity

One defining feature of the Delphi method is that it provides anonymity for each panel member. True anonymity has been defined when no one (including the researcher) can link a response to a respondent (Couper, 1984; Polit & Hunger, 1995). Thus, each member can express their opinions and views freely without feeling psychologically pressured, an issue which can arise in face-to-face meetings. Subject bias is therefore eliminated, as respondents are not known to one another (Goodman, 1986; Jeffery *et al.*, 1995), thus resulting in open and truthful responses.

Despite being cited as a key advantage of the Delphi technique, anonymity can also be viewed as a weakness, as it may result in non-disclosure (Hill & Fowles, 1975; Weicher, 2007) and respondents' not taking responsibility for their results (Sackman, 1975). Moreover, it may result in deindividuation limiting the 'extent to which exploratory thinking is possible' (Bowles, 1999, p. 32), thus removing 'the stimulation and spawning of ideas' (Rudy, 1996, p. 19). Indeed, some claim it results in isolation among panellists leading to some experiencing difficulties in their ability to clearly communicate their ideas so that others will understand them (Rotondi & Gustafson, 1996). In response, Sandrey and Bulger (2008) suggested reduced anonymity, such as biographical sketches of panel members shared before the Delphi commences, team-building techniques and straw-model construction be introduced to decrease isolation and increase communication in the Delphi process. However, the implications of utilising any of these approaches in the Delphi process, participation or outcomes are unknown.

Claims that the full anonymity can be assured in Delphi studies have been challenged on two main fronts. Firstly, as individual feedback is fed back to respondents, the researcher will know the panel members and their responses. Secondly, as the Delphi seeks to include experts, it often results in panel members knowing one another to the extent that individual responses can be attributed to a given member. Such challenges have led some authors (Rauch, 1979; McKenna, 1994a) to adopt the term quasi-anonymity (first suggested by Rauch, 1979) to refer to the fact that participants may know each other but their contributions to the study can remain anonymous. Rauch (1979) and Keeney *et al.* (2001) believed this membership of an elite expert club, where members do not meet but know one another may act as a motivator for participation. However, as Keeney *et al.* (2001) pointed out the consequence of a lack of full anonymity on Delphi findings is unclear as it is unknown if respondents change their opinion based on new information, or if indeed they do feel pressurised to conform to the groups majority, leading to what Gutierrez (1989) refers to as 'artificial consensus' (p. 33).

Expert 'opinion'

Whilst critical to the success of a Delphi, there are several difficulties associated with the selection of Delphi panellists. These include the terminology applied, identifying who an expert is, determining a panel's degree of expertise and the sampling procedure adopted to select panel members.

Traditionally, the term 'expert' has been used to describe participants in a Delphi study. However, the concept and term 'expert' is heavily contested in the Delphi literature (Bedford, 1972; Linstone & Turofff, 1975; Sackman, 1975; Williams & Webb, 1994a, 1994b; Hasson *et al.*, 2000; Baker *et al.*, 2006), yet some authors (Walker & Selfe, 1996; Crisp *et al.*, 1999; Mullen, 2003) claimed that there is a paucity of literature paid to the term. Nevertheless, in society there is a general acceptance of the concept of expert and expertise (Ayton, 1992), for example in a legal sense, expert evidence is normally admissible; however, psychological evidence challenges that acceptance (Sackman, 1975). It should, however, be noted that experts are not required for all Delphi's, Linstone (1978) suggested that a policy Delphi needs to include the general public at large while Turoff (1970) believed that in policy Delphi, advocates not experts are required. Therefore, a degree of flexibility is required when identifying expertise pertinent to Delphi studies.

The second challenge is identifying who an expert is. In 1971, Kaplan wrote, 'Throughout the Delphi literature, the definition of [Delphi panel members] has remained ambiguous' (p. 24). Despite this being written over 39 years ago, it still bears truth today. As early as 1971, Pill suggested that an 'expert' should be defined as anyone with a relevant input. This definition has essentially remained the same with slight word variation. For example, early definition refers to someone who 'has at his disposal a large store of background knowledge and a cultivated sensitivity to its relevance which permeates his intuitive insight' (Brown, 1968, p. 13). Later an expert was viewed as 'someone who has knowledge about a specific subject' (Keeney *et al.*, 2001, p. 196) used by Davidson *et al.* (1997), Lemmer (1998) and Green *et al.* (1999). McKenna (1994b) recommends the term an 'informed individual' (p. 1221), or as 'informed advocates' (Goodman, 1987, p. 730). Adler and Ziglio (1996) have added to this by outlining four requirements for expertise including:

1. Knowledge and experience with the issues under investigation
2. Capacity and willingness to participate
3. Sufficient time to participate
4. Effective communication skills

However, Sumsion (1998) and Bowling (1997) warned that the loose application of the term expert may result in the inclusion of individuals who have knowledge in a topic but not viewed as 'professionally expert' nor be representative of the total population targeted. For example, Crisp *et al.* (1999) suggested registered professional qualifications may not be consistent with expertise. For example, a nurse may know the practical difficulties on the ward of delivering care; but they may not know how to identify research priorities. Therefore, knowledge may not be consistent with expertise. Alternatively, experts may be selected on the basis of experience, such as the number of years worked in an area (Hardy *et al.*,

2004), but this may not make them an expert, as they may not posses the necessary knowledge or skills required (Baker *et al.*, 2006). Consequently, Crisp *et al.* (1999) suggested that, as few panels consist of true experts, the term 'informed advocates' be used instead. Indeed, some authors (Goodman, 1987; McKenna, 1994a) claimed experts in a Delphi is a misleading label which only enhances an illusionary concept, which Sackman (1975) warned this could lead to a 'pervasive expert halo effect' (p. 704) attributing excessive credence to Delphi results. Nguyen *et al.* (2009) also warned of the sole reliance on expert panels' results, specifically with regard to studies involving marginalised or socially sensitive behaviours. In their study, they found that despite using key informants, participants were only confident in 4 out of the 28 questions asked of them; therefore, they warn that basing credence or practice changes on the results of a Delphi needs to be approached with caution.

Without a clear definition, how then does one assess the suitability of an expert? In an attempt to define, identify and justify an expert, two key approaches have been adopted in the field, self-assessment and sample criteria. Suggested by Brown and Helmer (1964), numerous studies have asked for panel members to self-rate themselves, for example Bender *et al.* (1969) asked participants to outline their knowledge of each area based on awareness, reading or working. While, Linstone (1978) asked panellists to self-evaluate their familiarity with each item as fair, good or excellent, later Ishikawa *et al.* (1993) asked respondents to grade their expertise on each question on a 0–10 scale. Later, Dransfeld *et al.* (2000) reviewed each expert's experience, position in the company and the position of the company in industry as well as self-ranking for each response. However, a number of authors (Bender *et al.*, 1969; Catling & Rodgers, 1971; Rowe *et al.*, 1991; Mullen, 2003) have expressed their dissatisfaction with this self-weighting based on the fact that 'different people have very different ways of rating their own expertise' (Pill, 1971, p. 62). In addition, Rowe *et al.* (1991) pointed out that expertise should be established before the Delphi commences not during it. Moreover, Baker *et al.* (2006) highlighted little research has explored the differences between experts' responses who have rated themselves high and low.

Nonetheless, Mitchell (1991) widely advocated this approach as he believed it lead to accurate results indeed; some studies have reported that bias resulting from self-selection is unfounded. For example, McKee *et al.* (1991) compared the characteristics of medical consultants who participated in a Delphi panel and those who did not. Evidence showed only one difference between the two groups, a lower acceptance from consultants based in teaching hospitals, which the authors attributed to difficulties in accessing this sample's details. Whilst recognising the self-rating debate Van Zolingen and Klaassen (2003) suggest alternative approaches to self-rating may prove worthwhile, for example disregarding answers that come from people who rate themselves low on an item or place greater statistical weight on this answers that have come from high-rated participants. Another compromise suggested entails only asking for self-expertise on vital questions (von der Gracht, 2008). It is unclear, however, if such approaches have been utilised and the effect on this may have on process or outcomes.

The second approach towards identifying experts is the selection on the basis of specified criteria, normally derived from the purpose of the study. For example, on the basis of peer judgements, number of publications, educational status and positions held (Fisher, 1978). A number of studies have outlined how they have determined eligibility for inclusion, for example Miller (2001) required experts to be informed academics and/or consultants who have published in the area of sustainability in the last 2 years in one of the four major journals. Some studies have included vague criteria, such as on the basis of membership without defining what this means, or have specified a willingness and ability to take part (Goodman, 1987). Applying vague criteria increases the potential for researcher bias to be introduced (Rowe & Wright, 1999; van Zolingen & Klaassen, 2003; Hanafin, 2004) as a reliance on selecting only those respondents who are easily available, who researchers know have a reputation and who meet minimal criteria may result. Other studies, however, have left the reader guessing what, if any, criteria has been applied. For example, Wang *et al.* (2003) stated that the 'majority of the Chinese panel experts were identified by the study team, while most of the international experts were chosen with the help of the Ford Foundation reproductive health programme officers' (Wang *et al.*, 2003, p. 218), offering no insight into the criteria employed. The adoption of criteria needs to be justified or demonstrated to be associated with the genuine population understudy, to help enhance generalisability of the Delphi findings (Hicks, 1999).

Another criticism of the Delphi surrounds the issue of poor selection methodologies. The implication is that the Delphi does not depend on a statistical sample (Powell, 2003); therefore, representative sampling techniques are not appropriate (Beretta, 1996). Instead, representativeness is based upon the assessed qualities of the expert panel, rather than panel size. Consequently, more often than not, non-probability sampling techniques, including purposeful, convenience, criterion or snowballing sampling have been chosen. However, William and Webb (1994) have criticised the lack of random sampling procedures being used in Delphi studies. Many dismiss these concerns; however, what should be adopted remains vague.

Finally, Sackman (1975) suggested that there is little difference between findings from expert and non-expert panels, particularly in relation to evaluating social phenomena or forecasting, a claim rejected by Pill (1971). Some studies have investigated this, for example Jolson and Rossow (1971) and Rowe *et al.* (1991) both found increased accuracy over Delphi rounds for expert groups rather than non-expert panels. While, Walker

(1994) compared two panels comprising of physiotherapist researchers and newly qualified physiotherapists, and reported similar findings between the two panels. Leading Walker (1994) to question the level of expertness required in a Delphi.

The identification, selection and commitment of an expert in a Delphi study are regarded as the 'lynchpin of the method' (Green *et al.*, 1999, p. 200). However, the concept and process of including experts in a Delphi is complex. As stated by Sumsion (1998) 'there is no ready answer and it becomes the responsibility of each researcher to choose the most appropriate group of experts and defend that choice' (p. 154).

Level of consensus

It is a common misconception that the goal of a Delphi is used only to gain consensus, in reality it may not be possible or be the aim of the study. However, if the aim of the Delphi study is to obtain consensus, the definition of acceptable level of consensus to attain is contentious, and often this is an arbitrary figure, stated *post hoc* (Williams & Webb, 1994b) or entirely omitted in many Delphi studies (Powell, 2003). Without any guidance consensus has been defined, or claimed to be achieved in a variety of ways, for example:

- Aggregate the judgements of respondents (Delbecq *et al.*, 1975)
- Generating a pre-determined level of consensus (Williams & Webb, 1994b)
- Application of the subjective level of central tendency (Dajani *et al.*, 1979)
- Measuring the consistency of responses between successive rounds (Dajani *et al.*, 1979)

Each of these approaches has been debated, for example the attainment of a certain level of agreement (or majority rule) has been regarded as a measurement of consensus. Although as noted by Powell (2003) this is constructed at different levels, for example Williams and Webb (1994b) opted for 100% agreement for items, 95% (Stewart *et al.*, 1999), 80% (Putman *et al.*, 1995; Green *et al.*, 1999), 75% (Keeney *et al.*, 2006) to 51% (Loughlin & Moore, 1979). However, the process of how to decide upon a consensus level has been questioned by Crisp *et al.* (1997) who suggested the stability of the response through a series of rounds is a more reliable indicator of consensus. Therefore, less variance is understood to mean greater consensus (Rowe & Wright, 1999). However, this approach has also been subject to controversy (Hanafin, 2004) as a major criticism relates to its tendency to produce a false appearance of consensus among the respondents (Stewart, 1987) as a decrease in variance can be a consequence of attrition (Bardecki, 1984). Therefore, the pursuit of consensus can conceal important variations in views. For example, Rudy (1996) believed that 'extreme opinions will be masked by the statistical analysis' (p. 19) as panellists who hold such views are more likely to drop out than participants with more moderate views (Bardecki, 1984). Therefore, just because consensus has been reached should not imply that the correct answer has been found (Pill, 1971; Keeney *et al.*, 2001) a fact that most Delphi practitioners agree upon.

In 1975, Scheibe *et al.* criticised the use of statistical summaries as a measure of stability believing that it would not reflect resistance accurately. Despite this claim, various statistical tests have been applied to report a move towards consensus, such as standard deviation (Greatorex & Dexter, 2000), chi-square (Dajani *et al.*, 1979) and median (Brooks, 1979). However, selecting the most appropriate statistical measure to adopt has caused confusion in the literature (Murphy *et al.*, 1998). The statistical analysis of the Delphi is discussed in Chapter 6.

There are also a number of other issues relating to consensus that need to be considered. Firstly, how best to handle outliers or minority opinion, an issue which is often neglected. Donohoe and Needham (2008) recommended that researchers mitigate this risk by addressing and monitoring outliers and minority opinion. Secondly, as the Delphi does not allow for participants to elaborate upon their choices or ideas, critics warn that consensus is weakened (Walker & Selfe, 1996). Indeed, it cannot be assumed that the expert selected has actually completed the questionnaire themselves or has discussed it with others before being returned (Beretta, 1996). Finally, it is unclear how the Delphi actually contributes to shift towards consensus. Is it on the basis of new information or social pressure (Dalkey, 1967; Chan, 1982; Whitman, 1990; Munier & Ronde, 2001), factors which need further exploration.

Overall within Delphi literature, issues relating to identifying and measuring consensus is heatedly debated, with no clear answer advocated. Further research in this area is clearly required.

Limitations of the Delphi

Pressures of conformity

Often cited as a key advantage, it is assumed the Delphi does not fall foul to problems of groupthink and dominant personalities, which can lead to pressure for conformity and thus poor group decision-making (Fisher, 1978; Veal, 1992; Moeller & Shafer, 1994). However, contradictory evidence has suggested that Delphi members are exposed to strong group pressure to conform (Stewart, 1987; Woudenberg, 1991) with panel members facing the potential to fall victim to the band wagon effect (Geist, 2009). A number of authors have presented evidence that social-psychological factors can influence Delphi results (Sackman, 1975; Bardecki, 1984) leading to experts with divergent views either conforming to or abandoning the process (Rowe & Wright, 1999).

For example, Bardecki (1984) found that respondents who completed a Delphi study may not represent those who began it and that the impression of consensus may be partly due to attrition. Indeed, it has been found that when panellists are given fictitious or distorted feedback between iterations, they confirm their rating according to the false information (Cyphert & Gant, 1970; Scheibe *et al.*, 1975; Francis, 1977). In an early study Cyphert and Gant (1970) manipulated the data to see if they could alter consensus among an expert group. They chose an item which respondents had given a negative rating to and distorted the results to make it appear positive. Reasons given by panellists for the low rating were altered and reported back to the respondents as reasons for rating it high. The final consensus on the item, which had initially been very low, was well above average. Therefore, those who equate consensus with validity (Stewart, 1987), or truth need to tread carefully as it may only represent a 'collective bias rather than wisdom' (Chan 1982 p. 440).

Demanding nature of the technique

A common misconception is that a Delphi is a quick, cheap fix (Jones *et al.*, 1992; Everett, 1993). However, others have viewed it as a time-consuming, administratively complex, highly labour intensive and expensive process (Gordon & Helmer, 1964; Huckfeldt & Judd, 1974; Williams & Webb, 1994b; Fitzsimmons & Fitzsimmons, 2001; Zinn *et al.*, 2001; Yousuf, 2007a, 2007b) requiring considerable attention and effort from researchers and participants alike. The Delphi, unlike other forms of survey collection tools, requires ongoing time and attention commitment from participants.

It is claimed that the Delphi is not a successful decision-making tool, due to the time-consuming nature of the process (Jeffery *et al.*, 1995). Indeed, Donohoe and Needham (2008) considered the time required to complete a Delphi as a methodological disadvantage. Clearly, the labour and time intensity of a Delphi is linked to the number of rounds employed, time delays between rounds and the length of each round. Commonly, the number of rounds a Delphi adopts is restricted to two to three; however, evidence suggests that they can vary from two to ten rounds (Clark & Friedman, 1982; Errfmeyer *et al.*, 1986; Lang, 1994). Indeed, as many as 25 rounds in one Delphi study have been reported in the literature (Whitman, 1990). Time delays between rounds have also been proved to be problematic especially Sandrey and Bulger (2008) claim if the panel consists of non-professional or young respondents. The length of a Delphi places many demands and can directly affect the participant's motivation and choices identified (Whitman, 1990) and may account for the high dropout rates in some studies. Attrition has been found to occur mostly in the first round with numbers increasing as the Delphi progresses (van Zolingen &

Klaassen, 2003). However, limited research has explored the likelihood of participation or of dropout among certain expert groups.

Moreover, the demanding nature of the Delphi and lessons learned in the field by researchers have been reported (Green *et al.*, 1999; Keeney *et al.*, 2006). Although the application of the Delphi is widespread, Landeta (2006) reports it often has a negative image as a 'troublesome' technique (p. 469) which can be attributed to researchers using the method without fully comprehending the work and difficulty involved in its execution. Indeed, misunderstandings of the Delphi technique have resulted in critics and proponents alike highlighting the sloppy conduct of many studies. Criticising the way panellists have been selected or defined (Hill & Fowles, 1975; Preble, 1983) the wording of rounds (Hill & Fowles, 1975; Linstone, 1975), the large number of topics or questions per Delphi (Huckfeldt & Judd, 1974) and the superficial analysis of responses (Linstone, 1975).

Panel members may also report negative experience of participating in a Delphi study as a direct result of a lack of understating about the process, time and work commitment required (Hanafin, 2005; Landeta, 2006). Being subjected to answering the same question time again, with minimal or no interaction among members and participation reduced to statistical summaries, can be testing for anyone. Yet exploring and attempting to improve the Delphi experience from the panellists' viewpoint has received scant attention, an area which clearly requires further exploration.

Key learning points

- The paradigmatic assumption upon which a Delphi study is based is unclear; consequently many studies neglect to address this issue.
- Ironically, some of the advantages of the Delphi are also its disadvantages.
- A Delphi is only as good as the panel members it includes; however, no firm guidance exists regarding the size, composition and selection of participants.
- Commonly the selection of experts is based on either self-assessment or sampling criteria, with both approaches heavily criticised in literature.
- While the Delphi professes to provide anonymity, in reality this cannot be fully guaranteed, causing some to adopt the term 'quasi-anonymity'.
- Not all Delphi's aim to gain consensus.
- The definition or acceptable level of consensus to obtain is contentious and often arbitrary.
- A Delphi study is not an easy quick fix in reality: it is time-consuming, labour intensive and an expensive process.
- The consequence of the lack of anonymity and resulting social pressure is unknown and requires further exploration.

Recommended further reading

Goodman, C.M. (1987) The Delphi technique: a critique. *Journal of Advanced Nursing* 12, 729–734.

Helmer, O. (1963) *The Systematic Use of Expert Judgment in Operations Research.* The Rand Corporation, Santa Monica, California, p. 2795.

Keeney, S., Hasson, F. & McKenna, H.P. (2001) A critical review of the Delphi technique as a research methodology for nursing. *International Journal of Nursing Studies* 38, 195–200.

Sackman, H. (1975) *Delphi Critique.* Lexington Books, Massachusetts, Lexington.

Von der Gracht, H.A. (2008) *The Future of Logistics: Scenarios for 2025.* Gabler Edition Wissenschaft, Germany.

3 Applications of the Delphi in Nursing and Health Research

Introduction

Since the Delphi methods inception over 80 years ago, it has become an established methodological approach. Whilst not exclusively associated with any particular discipline, it has been extensively applied in a number of diverse fields including marketing, tourism, industry, politics, arts, education and health care. This chapter will evaluate its application in nursing and health research, especially in the area of identifying clinical nursing research priorities. The development and use of the technique from early applications to present day in nursing and health care will be traced and examples of how the technique has been adapted and the benefits of the method to this specialism have been discussed. Examples of good practice will be illustrated and an indicator of current interest provided.

Historical application of the Delphi technique in nursing

The Delphi technique was first mentioned by Whitehead in 1925, and then in 1948 by Churchman, both of whom called for the method to be viewed upon as a science 'for the use of expert judgment and as a simulation in areas where a complete theoretical framework was not available' (Lindeman, 1975, p. 435). However, it was not until later that the technique was adopted as an experiment.

In a review of the literature from the 1950s to 1980s, Rieger (1986) mapped the developmental stages of the Delphi method (see Table 3.1). The first stage, termed secrecy and obscurity, refers to the adoption of the technique by the RAND (Research ANd Development) Corporation, a research institution, founded by the United States Army Air, Forces and the Douglas Aircraft Company in 1946, whose initial remit was to research issues relating to national security. Two years later the Corporation changed to become an independent non-profit organisation focusing on the issues relating to national security, education, public welfare

The Delphi Technique in Nursing and Health Research, First Edition, © S. Keeney, F. Hasson and H. McKenna   Published 2011 by Blackwell Publishing Ltd.

Table 3.1   Rieger's (1986) five developmental stages of the Delphi technique

Stage	Time-frame	Definition	Study example
Secrecy and obscurity	1950s to early 1960s	Focus on sensitive issues, such as military intelligence operations	Seminal study, estimating Soviet bombing scheduled in the US locations (Dalkey & Helmer, 1962). Research dominated by RAND methodology
Novelty	Mid to late 1960s	Long-range forecasting tool applied in industry and human services	Seminal study, forecast trends some 50 years into the future on six key domains: scientific breakthroughs, population growth, automation, space progress, probability and prevention of war and future weapon systems trends (Gordon & Helmer, 1964)
Popularity	Late 1960s to Mid 1970s	Estimated threefold increase in Delphi study activity over previous stage (Listone & Turoff, 1975) of studies employing the technique in a range of disciplines	Predictions about future events in nursing education were undertaken (Burnside & Lenburg, 1970; Mussallem, 1970; Bramwell & Hykawy, 1974; Stead-Lorenzo, 1975) The broader utility of the Delphi was first recognised by nursing profession by Lindeman (1974, 1975) exploring clinical nursing research priorities
Scrutiny	1970–1980	Methodological critique of the problems and issues arising from research	Welty (1971), Pill (1971), Sackman (1975) and Murray (1979); critique the delphi resulting with a continual heated discourse in the literature
Continuity and reflection	1980-present	Delphi is accepted as a legitimate methodological approach	Continuity of its use in nursing and health-related field and critiques of the approach in health-related literature appeared (McKenna, 1994a; Keeney et al., 2001; Mullen, 2003; Powell, 2003)

and scientific causes. In 1948, the Corporation adopted and applied the Delphi method as an experiment, based upon earlier work which high-lighted the superiority of collective expert opinion over individual (Kaplan et al., 1949; Helmer & Rescher, 1959).

The first in-house study employed the Delphi process to help predict horse race outcomes in 1948, statisticians found that individuals would lose on a number of races; however, they would not lose as much when following group opinions of the pooled handicappers. However, as Quade (1967) later explained 'although the experiment showed promise criticism of its subject matter and some obvious defects set the effort back ten years or so' (p. 4). In 1951, referred to as PROJECT-Delphi, Norman Crolee Dalkey and Olaf Helmer-Hirschberg, undertook an experiment to 'apply expert opinion to the selection, from the viewpoint of a Soviet strategic planner, of an optimal US industrial target system and to the estimation of the number of A-bombs required to reduce the munitions output by a prescribed amount' (Dalkey & Helmer, 1962, p. 1). Put simply, they aimed to gain consensus on 'the probable effects of a massive atomic bombing attack on the United States' (Helmer, 1975, p. xix); however, for reasons of security the results of this experiment were not published until 1962 (see Dalkey & Helmer, 1962).

Building upon early work, the second stage novelty, saw a shift in attention towards non-military issues, for example Helmer and Quade (1963) proposed the application of the technique in economic planning of developing countries. However, the most notable work during this period was undertaken by Ted Gordon in conjunction with Olaf Helmer, whose research focused upon long-range forecasts. Representing the first real large-scale application of the method Gordon and Helmer (1964) asked 82 professionals, to identify future developments and the probable effects in six areas, namely scientific breakthroughs, population growth, automation, space progress, probability and prevention of war and future weapon systems trends. Whilst recommended (Seyffer, 1965; Applund, 1966) no early studies adopting the Delphi to predict future events in nursing were undertaken (Bramwell & Hykawy, 1974); indeed, it was not until the next chapter that the true utility of the Delphi method was recognised within the health care domain.

The third developmental stage of the Delphi entitled, popularity, occurred during the late 1960s to mid 1970s, which saw the adoption of the method in an array of specialisms including medicine and nursing. The adaptability of the Delphi was exploited to assess experts' judgments in a number of ways, for example forecasting and priority setting. A number of early research projects adopted the method to predict future events in medicine developments (Bender et al., 1969), disease patterns (Longhurst, 1971), nursing education (Burnside & Lenburg, 1970; Mussallem, 1970; Bramwell & Hykawy, 1974; Stead-Lorenzo, 1975), nursing services (McNally, 1974) and manpower planning (GMENAC, 1980).

For example, funded by Smith, Kline & French Laboratories in the United States, Bender et al. (1969) employed the Delphi to predict the developments in biomedical research, diagnosis, medical therapy, health care and medical education. He asked panellists to envisage what they thought may happen in each area over the next 50 years. Findings from this early study helped to develop a 5-year work plan.

The Delphi was also used to forecast disease patterns, for example Longhurst (1971) used a three-round Delphi to predict how changes in nutrition, income and prenatal care would impact on birth weight and intellectual development of young children; Longhurst (1971) provided experts with real data to identify factors that could influence outcomes and the extent to which this may occur. Results from this study enabled cost-benefit analysis of government services aimed at pregnant women and young children.

The method was also used during the 1970s to predict developments in nursing education, for example in Canada, Bramwell and Hykawy (1974) drew on the expertise of 13 nurse teachers (either in university, clinical or government agency setting) to predict future occurrences in the field of nurse education and when they would occur. Four rounds were conducted with panellists, the first round required experts to list 10 predictions in the next 50 years, which were collapsed into 38 statements. In Round 2 panellists were asked to speculate the time interval that these events were likely to occur in. It was not until Round 3 that predictions plus group responses for each statement was feedback and, if a response was different from the group, they were asked to justify their view. The final round required experts to review the group responses once again along with recording their reactions to the Delphi technique which produced a mix response, with some suggesting it helped to stimulate thinking while others were frustrated due to the lack of engagement with colleagues.

An example of predicting manpower needs is illustrated by a study in the United States, by the Graduate Medical Education National Advisory Committee (GMENAC – now the Department and Health and Human Services) undertaken in 1976 but published in 1980. Using a modified Delphi, the GMENAC designed specialty-specific expert panels including practicing and academic physicians with nurse practitioners and physician assistants, to identify the future physician requirements for the United States. The Committee predicted a surplus of 70 000 physicians by the year 2000, recommending immediate reductions of graduate numbers into medical schools. Whilst considered one of the most detailed studies of the time (Morgan, 1982), it was fundamentally flawed as it did not ask panellists to consider other types of health care professionals required; therefore, the numbers of physicians thought required were artificially inflated.

During the popularity stage the broader application and development of the Delphi technique was recognised in the nursing and health care domain. Lindeman (1974, 1975) is cited as one of the first nursing professionals to have employed the approach to identify clinical nursing research priorities and since her work many others have followed suit. Crisp *et al.* (1999) attribute Lindeman's work to having greatly influenced the application of the technique in nursing, citing the ongoing use of the method to identify research priorities and to have encouraged the Delphi to become accepted within nursing research. During this time, the versatility of the Delphi was also used to identify community health care needs (Schoeman & Mahajan, 1977), curriculum development (Spivey, 1971; Hope, 1977), interpretation of research findings (Milholland *et al.*, 1973); assessment of research and development projects (Derian & Morize, 1973), identification of competencies (Sims, 1979) and towards the development of an index of hospital performance measures (Grimes & Moseley, 1976).

The third stage of the Delphi's development scrutiny, Rieger (1986) noted a change in the literature towards the in-depth methodological scrutiny of the approach. One of the most notable and widely cited critiques was undertaken by Sackman in 1975, then an employee of the RAND Corporation. The majority of literature critiquing the method was undertaken outside the health care domain. Indeed, it was not until the final stage, continuity and reflection, when papers critiquing the technique started to appear in the health-related literature (e.g. Goodman, 1987; McKenna, 1994a; Williams & Webb, 1994b; Crisp *et al.*, 1999; Keeney *et al.*, 2001; Mullen, 2003; Powell, 2003).

Whilst recognizing the methodological flaws of the Delphi, Donohoe and Needham (2008) note a sixth stage in the Delphi's development, towards application and refinement, with attention being placed upon developing guidelines for Delphi practitioners (Eggers & Jones, 1998; Hasson *et al.*, 2000; Keeney *et al.*, 2006; Skulmoski *et al.*, 2007). Whilst the development of such standards is ongoing and criticisms continue, the utilisation of the Delphi is increasing (McKenna, 1994a; Moseley & Mead, 2001; Thangaratinam & Redman, 2005), especially in nursing and health care, as the examples in Table 3.2 illustrate.

Since the Delphi's development, it has been widely utilised although refinements in its methodology are ongoing. Whilst the five developmental stages identified by Rieger (1986) provide some indication of the techniques progress, the future of the method is uncharted with more chapters potentially ahead.

Identification of clinical nursing research priorities

In the nursing literature, many applications of the Delphi technique have been reported in the literature, one of the most common has been to identify nursing research priorities (Daniels & Ascough, 1999; McKenna & Keeney, 2008a). Research priority setting is widely advocated to assist researchers and to ensure the alignment of funding with national evidence needs (Working Group on Priority Setting, 2000) whilst enhancing practice outcomes and policy (Drennan *et al.*, 2007).

The technique has been frequently used to establish priorities for many specialist practice (see Table 3.3) and has been used in other health-related disciplines, such as occupational health (Sadhra *et al.*, 2001), physiotherapy (Soma *et al.*, 2009) and health informatics (Brender *et al.*, 2000) for similar purposes. Studies employing the Delphi have been used to set national research and development priorities with a direct view to influence policy for nursing in the UK (Scott *et al.*, 1999). Others have been undertaken to establish research priorities for nursing organisations, for example the

Table 3.2   Applications of the Delphi method in nursing and health care

Application of the Delphi method	Example study
Clinical problems	Rauch *et al.* (2009) validated the 'comprehensive International Classification of Functioning, Disability and Health (ICF) Core Set for Rheumatoid Arthritis (RA)' amongst 57 experienced RA nurses, using a three-round Delphi technique. Panellists were asked about patients' problems, resources and environment aspects; nurses are responsible for and results were linked to ICF components. Results indicate majority support for the ICF guidelines from nurses
Funding and service requirements (priorities)	Wilson and Opolski (2009) evaluated stakeholder views on the dissemination of a cardiovascular computerised decision support system (CDSS) program among 11 experts. They adopted a two-round modified Delphi technique, incorporating a review of the literature and semi-structured interviews. Financial incentives followed by joint promotion with a professional agency were most highly rated
Disease patterns (forecasting) health technology	Leang (2008) reviewed 25 public health physicians' opinions on the impact and future demands of HIV/Aids on Cambodia health services. Panellists were asked to solicit and rank ways in which HIV was likely to impact upon health services through a two-round Delphi. Mother-to-child transmission issues, demand on services and health prevention and promotion strategies were ranked highly
Education	Dewolfe *et al.* (2010) used a modified two-round Delphi to gain consensus among preceptors of nursing students on recruitment, support and retention. Focus groups were also undertaken to explore those issues which did not obtain agreement upon. Results suggest recruitment strategies should emphasise personal satisfaction, and agreement was recorded on ways to support students in placement
Policy	McKeown and Gibson (2007) using a two-round Delphi determined the political influence and profile of 40 nurses working in the area of hepatitis C. Results indicate the need for structural and policy changes to ensure nurses are included

American Association of Critical Care Nurses (Lindquist *et al.*, 1993) or the Society for Urologic Nursing (Demi *et al.*, 1996). In addition, the Delphi method has also been used to establish priorities for specific conditions, such as HIV/AIDS (Sowell, 2000), low back pain (Henschke *et al.*, 2007), infection control (Lynch *et al.*, 2001) and surgical infection (Nathens *et al.*, 2006) to name but a few.

One of the earliest studies using the Delphi to clinically identify priorities in nursing was undertaken in the United States, by Lindeman in 1975. Using a conventional four-round Delphi she sought the opinions of 433 nurse and non-nurse (i.e. administrators, clinicians, educators, funders, etc.) experts to identify 'burning questions about the practice of nursing' (p. 436). From the 433 panel initially recruited, 341 completed all four

Table 3.3   Specialist nursing areas research priorities setting: Delphi studies

Specialist practice areas	Delphi studies
Mental health	Ventura and Waligora-Serafin (1981), Wilkinson and Williams (1985), Davidson *et al.* (1997), Naylor *et al.* (2008), Owens *et al.* (2008)
Palliative care	Cawley and Webber (1995), Chang and Daly (1998), Daniels and Howlett (2001), Steele *et al.* (2008), Malcolm *et al.* (2009)
Cancer nursing	Oberst (1978), Hinds *et al.* (1990), Stetz *et al.* (1995), Rudy *et al.* (1998), Daniels and Ascough (1999), Fochtman and Hinds (2000), Soanes *et al.* (2000), Barrett *et al.* (2001), Browne *et al.* (2002), McIlfatrick and Keeney (2003), Grundy and Ghazi (2009)
Public health nursing	Albrecht and Perry (1992), Misener *et al.* (1997), Brooks and Barrett (2003), Madigan and Vanderboom (2005), Hauck *et al.* (2007)
Administration	Henry *et al.* (1987), Lynn *et al.* (1998)
Critical care	Lewandowski and Kositsky (1983), Lindquist *et al.* (1993), Cronin and Owsley (1993), Heffline *et al.* (1994), Daly *et al.* (1996), Lopez (2003), Jurkovich *et al.* (2004), Mamaril *et al.* (2009)
Paediatric nursing	Hinds *et al.* (1994), Broome *et al.* (1996), Schmidt *et al.* (1997), Monterosso *et al.* (2001), Ota *et al.* (2008), Byrne *et al.* (2008)
Vascular nursing	Hatton and Nunnelee (1995), Lewis *et al.* (1999)
Orthopaedic nursing	Salmond (1994), Sedlak *et al.* (1998)
Urologic nursing	Demi *et al.* (1996)
Respiratory	Sheikh *et al.* (2008)
School nursing	Edwards (2002)
Neurology	Koopman *et al.* (1995)
Emergency nursing	Bayley *et al.* (1994), Bayley *et al.* (2004), Rodger *et al.* (2004)
Occupational health nursing	Rogers *et al.* (2000)

rounds. The initial open round resulted in over 2000 items being recorded which was reduced to 150 for Round 2. Priority was attributed towards measuring the quality of care, professional role of the nurse, the nursing and research process. Patient welfare issues such as interventions related to stress, care of the aged, pain and patient education, were also identified within the top 10%.

Since 1975, a number of studies have explored clinical nursing research priorities (see Table 3.4). A number of these studies have explored the nursing research priorities on a national scale, for example Northern England (Bond & Bond, 1982), Scotland (Macmillan *et al.*, 1989), Ireland (Drennan *et al.*, 2007), Spain (Moreno-Casbas *et al.*, 2001), Sweden (Bäck-Pettersson *et al.*, 2008), Hong Kong (French *et al.*, 2002); Korea (Kim *et al.*, 2002) and Australia (Jones *et al.*, 1989; Bartu *et al.*, 1991, 1993; Annells *et al.*, 1997, 2005; Bell *et al.*, 1997), while others have identified priorities for specific purposes, such as a recently merged health care system (Forte *et al.*, 1997) or for a specific health care trust (Kirkwood *et al.*, 2003).

Table 3.4   Clinical nursing research priorities: Delphi studies

Years	No.	Authors
1970–1980	1	Lindeman (1975)
1981–1990	5	Bond and Bond (1982), Goodman (1986), Dennis *et al.* (1989), Macmillan *et al.* (1989), Jones *et al.* (1989), Nappier *et al.* (1990)
1991–2000	10	Bartu *et al.* (1991), Fitzpatrick *et al.* (1991), Macilraith (1992), Alderson *et al.* (1992), Pinyeard *et al.* (1993), Bartu *et al.* (1993), Bell *et al.* (1997), Forte *et al.* (1997), Annells *et al.* (1997), Scott *et al.* (1999)
2001–2010	14	Moreno-Casbas *et al.* (2001), Kim *et al.* (2002, 2004), French *et al.* (2002), Kirkwood *et al.* (2003), Chang *et al.* (2003), Cohen *et al.* (2004), Annells *et al.* (2005), Fenwick *et al.* (2006), Drennan *et al.* (2007), Bäck-Pettersson *et al.* (2008), Butler *et al.* (2009), Wiener *et al.* (2009)

Whist the goal may be to establish research priorities; a review of the studies reveals the latitude exercised in the implementation of the Delphi, with regards, design, number of rounds and sample size. A number of these studies have been deliberately chosen to illustrate, the abovementioned issues will be reviewed, for example in the UK; Bond and Bond (1982) employed a three-round conventional Delphi to establish the clinical nursing research priorities among 271 nurses working in England. Respondents were asked to 'list not more than five questions or problems regarding clinical nursing' (p. 567). From a total of 271 participants, 214 responded to Round 1, 178 to Round 2 and 169 to Round 3. Findings reveal priority was attributed to items relating to leadership issues.

Later, Kim *et al.* (2004) explored priorities among a national sample of Korean nurses based in academic and clinical settings ($N = 347$). Using a modified two-round Delphi, panellists were asked to list five nursing research areas rated on three dimensions, the degree of nurses' lead role, contribution to the profession and health and welfare of patients. A total of 1013 areas were identified which were collapsed into 29 categories. Key priorities related to advanced practice nursing system, interventions, competency, quality and effectiveness of nursing care and standardisation. In addition, research on home health care, nurse training, older people and utilisation of findings were also cited as important.

In one of the largest studies to date, undertaken to explore research priorities, Drennan *et al.* (2007) undertook a large-scale three-round, decision Delphi and consultation workshops to identify, rate and set timescales for clinical, managerial and educational nursing research priorities. A total of 1695 Irish nurses were initially approached to take part in the Delphi with 122 nurses participating in discussion group workshops. In total, 24 priorities were recorded, many of which are similar to priorities identified in other European countries and North America. The top clinical issues related to outcomes of care delivery, staffing issues and communication. Managerial issues related to recruitment and retention and input into health policy and decision-making.

Finally, in Sweden, Bäck-Pettersson *et al.* (2008) used a three-round Delphi to survey 118 clinicians from various disciplines including nursing, teaching and administration to record vital areas for future patient-related nursing research and research areas based on clinical practice. Ninety-five panellists (81%) completed all rounds. Round 1 resulted in 380 areas being identified. Final priorities revealed research that enhances clinical practice; patient's well-being and a caring environment were illuminated.

In conclusion, a review of these studies indicates the array of international and national Delphi studies have been undertaken to explore clinical nursing research priorities. However, there is a lack of discussion on how results and Delphi designs compare. Such evidence could potentially inform the Delphi methods development and utility in the future in this area.

Trends of the Delphi in nursing

Since the 1970s, the usage of the Delphi method has exploded in the literature and much attention has been given towards analysing the trends in its use in a number of areas including tourism (Green *et al.*, 1990; Donohoe & Needham, 2008) education (Judd, 1972), public sector (Preble, 1983) and social sciences (Landeta, 2006). In the mid-1970s, Delbecq *et al.* (1975) and Linstone and Turoff (1975) published two seminal books that evaluated the technique and also provided examples of its application. Linstone and Turoff (1975) found 134 articles published on the Delphi prior to 1970 and another 355 published between 1970 and 1974. The majority of these articles were found in the field of psychology, sociology, economics, philosophy, planning, statistics and economics.

In 1977, Brockhaus and Michelsen in a study of 800 Delphi method studies concluded that the method was most applied in science and engineering, with only 50 undertaken in biological sciences and medicine. Both O'Brien (1979) and Rieger (1986) noted an interest in the application of the Delphi among doctoral dissertations particularly in education. Later Reid (1988) analysed the application of the Delphi and concluded that use of the technique in health research was limited. In a review of papers between 1975 and 1994 inclusive, Gupta and Clarke (1996) identified 463 papers dealing with the method and its application in research. Application of the Delphi was found in three main areas including education, business and health care. Building on this, Bowles (1999) identified 288 papers published between 1981 and 1998 but reported a diminishing interest in the approach in nursing and related areas after 1994, which was attributed to the methods costs and attractiveness. Similarly Mullen (2000) and de

Table 3.5   Frequency of Delphi papers published in Science Direct

Period	No. of articles
2004	29
2005	39
2006	47
2007	41
2008	53
2009	82
Total	291

Meyrick (2003) both noted diminishing interest towards the usage of the method in health care, with only six out of 125 papers between 1995 and 2001 nursing related (de Meyrick, 2003).

More recently, building on Gupta and Clarke (1996) work, Landeta (2006) reviewed the Delphi literature and revealed that 414 related articles had been published during 1995 and 1999, and 677 between 2000 and 2004, and noted a growing application in doctoral research studies. Although this study does not detail the specific application areas within which the Delphi was utilised, it does report an ongoing interest in the method.

Following on from this study, the extent of the use of the Delphi in the nursing and health care literature and trends over time were explored. Science Direct, database was reviewed using the following search terms, 'Delphi Technique' and 'Delphi Method' to appear in the title, abstract and keyword, in English language papers appearing from 2004 to 2009 inclusive. Table 3.5 outlines the number of articles published.

A total of 291 papers of typical examples within the health care area were identification of core competencies, research priorities, professional workload and roles and clinical guidelines.

In general, estimates of the use of the Delphi method in nursing and health-related services research are increasing from 300 (Bowles, 1999) to at least 1000 (McKenna, 1994a), to 1400 (Thangaratinam & Redman, 2005) to 2500 (NHS Institute for Innovation and Improvement, 2008), indicating that the technique has a firm and definite place in health care development.

Key learning points

- Nursing and health-related researchers were slow to adopt the Delphi technique as a suitable research procedure.
- Rieger (1986) identified five developmental stages of the method including secrecy and obscurity, novelty, popularity, scrutiny and continuity and reflection. An additional chapter refers to adaption and refinement of the method.

- Lindeman (1975) study represents a significant influence on the direction of research development in nursing.
- Since then there has been a growing acceptance and popularity of the Delphi within the nursing and health care arena.

Recommended further reading

Gupta, U.G. & Clarke, R.E. (1996) Theory and applications of the Delphi technique: A bibliography (1975–1994). *Technological Forecasting and Social Change* 53, 185–211.

Lindeman, C.A. (1975) Delphi survey of priorities in clinical nursing research. *Nursing Research* 24, 434–441.

Rieger, W.G. (1986) Direction in Delphi developments: dissertations and their quality. *Technological Forecasting and Social Change* 29, 195–204.

4 How to Get Started with the Delphi Technique

Introduction

The success with any research lies with effective planning. In theory, the Delphi process might appear straightforward; in practice, it is not. For a successful outcome, irrespective of Delphi type, a researcher must consider and plan the various steps associated with the technique before entering the field. This chapter outlines some of the key planning and execution activities for a Delphi, namely preparation, administration, mailing and content analysis.

Preparation and practicalities

The preparation considerations a researcher deliberates upon before employing the Delphi are rarely reported in the literature, yet paradoxically, this stage is one of the most important. There are a number of key issues which a researcher must consider before embarking on the Delphi process and they include the suitability of the Delphi, availability of resources and the definition and level of consensus to be applied. Each of these issues will now be discussed separately.

Suitability of the Delphi

The first key step a researcher must undertake is to identify the nature and scope of the problem to be explored; once this is stated consideration must be given towards the appropriateness of the Delphi method to address this problem. Turoff (1970) identified four situations when it would be appropriate to use the Delphi; these include exploring judgements; generating or correlating informed judgements and exposing diverse views. Later, Linstone and Turoff (1975) expanded this to include, when the research problem does not lend itself to precise analytical techniques but can benefit from subjective judgements, when the population is geographically and

The Delphi Technique in Nursing and Health Research, First Edition, © S. Keeney, F. Hasson and H. McKenna   Published 2011 by Blackwell Publishing Ltd.

professionally diverse and when logistical reasons (such as time and cost) would make frequent meetings unfeasible. Others maintain that the Delphi is suitable for areas where there is a lack of empirical data (Farrell & Scherer, 1983) or when instant decisions are not required (Beech, 1999). A Delphi exercise, however, can encompass any one or combination of these objectives; nevertheless, the key determinate in the selection is the nature of the research problem.

Availability of resources

Many researchers underestimate the skills, time and financial commitment required to undertake a Delphi, yet such issues underlie its success. As noted in the earlier chapters, the Delphi literature lacks sufficient guidelines for researchers to refer to, consequently difficult decisions will have to be faced without the aid of any empirical or professional guidance. Numerous researchers have reported upon the dilemmas and lessons learnt in the field (see Green et al., 1999; Biondo et al., 2008; Hung et al., 2008; Geist, 2009). Therefore, conducting a Delphi requires a researcher to be thoroughly familiar with the capabilities and limitations of the technique. In conjunction, a researcher needs to be proficient in the collection and analysis of both qualitative and quantitative data, possess excellent interpersonal and administration skills.

Let's repeat this as consideration of these skills is often underestimated or overlooked resulting in numerous problems. Before undertaking a Delphi study a researcher needs to know how a Delphi works, he/she must know how to manage and analyse data, how to deal with others, communicate effectively (written and verbal), lead, motivate and problem solve. In conjunction, he/she must have organisational, administration and analytical skills. Underestimate these at your peril!

Once you have considered the researchers' skills, you also need to think about the required capabilities of the target sample. Traditionally, a Delphi is administered using paper and pencil; however, this requires panellists to have literacy skills. Poor reading and writing skill was an issue Oranga and Nordberg (1993) faced in their Delphi study which resulted in interviewers being trained to assist panellists, completing questionnaires. However, with advanced technology, the increasing use of electronic communications requires computer literacy skills and access to such equipment. Moreover, regardless of the type of delivery chosen, as the Delphi unfolds panel members are often fed back analysis in the form of statistical summaries; consideration must also be given towards the skill the experts have to decipher this information. It cannot be assumed potential panel members possess these skills.

Undertaking a Delphi study is time-consuming, to allow for recruitment, rounds to be designed, distributed, returned, analysed and redesigned. Too often the period required for completing such a study is underestimated. While it is impossible to accurately predict exactly what will occur over the course of the research process, a detailed project timetable should be developed. One useful approach is to break down a Delphi project into smaller sections. For example, initial tasks might consist of ordering stationary, identifying participants, developing administration systems and gaining participants' consent. Just one of these tasks, gaining consent, is estimated to take up to 2–3 weeks (Price, 2005). Sufficient time should also be allocated for each round, estimates are available on how long a traditional postal round may take, for example between 3–4 weeks (Gordon, 1994; Eggers & Jones, 1998) and 6–8 weeks (Duffield, 1993; Beretta, 1996; Keeney et al., 2006). However, with technological advancement the administration and analysis time can be substantially reduced to days or weeks. Nevertheless, a researcher must remember a Delphi does take time and it is important to ensure sufficient time is built into a project timescale to enable the team to undertake robust research.

The cost of undertaking research projects can vary substantially; however, whilst a Delphi project is considered a cheaper alternative than face-to-face meetings, it still will incur costs. Consideration must be given towards budgeting for staff, printing, photocopying, telephone, stationary, postage and consumable costs. Public relation activities and awareness campaigns may also be needed. The cost of undertaking a Delphi is rarely reported, one study by Oranga and Nordberg (1993) estimated execution of their modified Delphi totalled US$3527 with the most expensive components being information feedback, data processing and panel recruitment. However, Cuhls et al. (2002) estimated an international Delphi cost 700 000 Euro in 1998, including the end report. Costs will obviously vary but consideration of these is important for any research study.

Level of consensus

If the aim of the Delphi study is to gain consensus, then deliberation must also be given towards deciding upon the level of consensus to be applied. Often, however, many Delphi studies employ arbitrary levels, state such figures *post hoc* at the data-analysis stage or rarely provide a definition of what constitutes consensus (Evans, 1997). There are different types of criteria for describing when consensus is reached; for example the two most commonly used are the statistical approach and percentage levels.

Statistical analyses, such as measures of central tendency mean (Murray & Jarman, 1987) and median and mode (Hasson et al., 2000) have been used to illustrate the collective judgements of respondents. However, Scheibe et al. (1975) criticised the use of percentage measures, suggesting the need to measure the stability of responses over successive rounds. Another way of defining consensus refers to a certain percentage of the vote's falls within prescribed range (Williams & Webb, 1994b; Miller, 2006).

Table 4.1   Preparation questions

1	What do you want or need to find out?
2	Does it require a form of group work?
3	Does the use of a Delphi make sense?
4	What skills does the researcher need?
5	What skills do panellists need?
5	What resources (time, money) do you have?
6	What is the definition and level of consensus to be adopted?

However, with no standard threshold for consensus this is a contentious issue with varying opinions littered in the Delphi literature, as to what constitutes an acceptable level. For example Loughlin and Moore (1979) suggest 51%, Boyce *et al.* (1993) set consensus at 66%; McKenna (1994a) in his review of the Delphi method suggests a 51% level, Green (1982) proposes 70% or higher, Mitchell (1991) and Keeney *et al.* (2006) propose 75% level acceptable, while Ulschak (1983) wants 80%. However, with no scientific rationale for selection, the key question is how is the level chosen? Keeney *et al.* (2006) suggest the use of confidence intervals may help to determine the cut-off point. For a researcher this decision needs to be based primarily on the aims and objectives of the study, with the realisation that the stricter the criteria the more difficult it is to obtain consensus (Fink *et al.*, 1984). Nevertheless, it is recommended that a researcher states the definition and level of consensus to be adopted prior to data collection.

Preparation for a Delphi study is vital, spending time on the initial stages of a project can help overcome some of the major problems and dilemmas a Delphi practitioner may face as the study progresses. Table 4.1 sets out some of the basic questions a researcher needs to raise before embarking on a Delphi investigation.

Identifying target sample – panel of experts

After the initial considerations, a researcher must decide on who participates in the study. As Duffield (1988) acknowledged, decisions concerning who to include in a Delphi study are by no means as straightforward as they appear to be when represented in the literature. Nevertheless, the Delphi is only as good as the experts who participate; therefore, if the identification and recruitment of the panel are questionable then the results of the study can also be queried. Regardless of Delphi type, there are a number of key sample issues for the researcher to consider, namely identifying the sample population, criteria, size, response and attrition rate.

Who is the target population?

The first step is to determine the target population of interest, that is who should be included in the study. Your choice of who to include will be influenced primarily by the nature of your research question. Whilst contentious, the participants in a Delphi are commonly referred to as 'experts' as it is assumed that they have more knowledge of the topic under investigation than most people. For example, Clayton (1997) suggests that an expert, not a general population, opinion is needed when attempting to define best practice for a particular medical procedure. Similarly, if investigating the role of the health visitor Lemmer (1998) recommends the inclusion of health visitors who have more knowledge about the topic area. While in policy or decision Delphi respondents' are those with a vested interest in the outcomes, such as decision-makers, key stakeholders or lobbyists, who have an authority to influence outcomes. In all research, the goal is to choose the best participants to provide the information; doing so may involve discussions about the relative advantages and disadvantages of different types of target populations, involved such as lay people or policy makers.

How do you select your experts?

Most research uses some form of sampling and Delphi studies are no different. The sample to include in a Delphi study will obviously vary according to the Delphi design selected and the purpose of the project (Jairath & Weinstein, 1994). There are a number of approaches adopted in the Delphi literature. For example, Thompson *et al.* (2004) used anonymous postal questionnaires as part of the Delphi, to a random sample of 300 members of the British Association of Sport and Exercise Medicine. However, in order to ensure the participation of the right kinds of experts, who understand the issues have a vision and represent a substantial variety of viewpoints (Czinkota & Ronkainen, 1997), sample selection in Delphi studies may not be random. Many Delphi studies have employed non-probability sampling techniques, used individually or in combination, such as convenience and snowballing to recruit the sample. For example, panel members have been identified through literature searches and/or recommendation from other recognised experts in the field (Gordon, 1992); such approaches are often adopted when the research population is hard to identify (Polit & Hungler, 1999). Whichever type of Delphi employed, the composition of the sample relates to the validity of the results of the research (Spencer-Cooke, 1989); therefore, considerable attention needs to be given to issues related to sampling and selection.

Sampling criteria

In order to avoid methodological pitfalls a researcher should adhere to stringent protocols for determining who qualifies as an 'expert'. Essentially, this is a list of characteristics essential for a participant to be included in the study or cause a person to be excluded from the study. The development of which will obviously depend upon the context in which the Delphi methodology is used.

To ensure the inclusion of a heterogeneous sample, a researcher can identify very board sampling criteria, such as any adult over the age of 18, willing to participate and can read and write English. However, most Delphi studies require a homogeneous sample to ensure the appropriate expert panel is included, for example health professionals must have 3 years post-qualification experience in the clinical area, be educated to postgraduate level, be employed in the clinical area and willing to participate. Novakowski and Wellar (2008) advocate that the use of strict selection criteria as they believe it can help to ensure high-quality responses but also means that the panellists themselves can feel validated by the experience. Nevertheless, the more focused the criteria the greater limits are placed upon the generalisation of the study's findings.

For the conventional and real-time Delphi, a number of authors have suggested a heterogeneous sample is used to ensure that the entire spectrum of opinion is determined (Starkweather et al., 1975; Moore, 1987; Synowiez & Synowiez, 1990). This can be achieved by including different panels of experts, such as doctors, nurses and health visitors. In contrast, for the policy and decision Delphi heterogeneity is not a concern, as the key would be the inclusion of pertinent stakeholders or decision-makers (Jairath & Weinstein, 1994).

A number of studies have explicitly stated their selection criteria (see Tables 4.2 and 4.3). Some studies have used geographical representatives (Biondo et al., 2008), professional and speciality of members (Huang et al., 2008), educational status and willingness to participate in the study (Evans, 1997). Some authors (Ziglio, 1996; Skulmoski et al., 2007) have identified generic criteria to guide researchers; these include the following:

- Knowledge and practical experience with the issue under investigation
- Capacity and willingness to contribute
- Assurance that sufficient time will be dedicated to the Delphi exercise
- Good written communication skills
- Experts' skills and knowledge need not necessarily be accompanied by standard academic qualifications or degrees

Regardless of what criteria are adopted, there is no ready answer. Nevertheless, it is the responsibility of each researcher to choose the most appropriate criteria for experts and to provide a rationale for that choice (Sumsion, 1998).

What size does the sample have to be?

There is no one sample size advocated for Delphi studies. The literature provides a wide range of possibilities, for example Novakowski and

Table 4.2 Examples of open Round 1

Author and year	Delphi focus	Delphi type and round number	Sample	Sample criteria	Round 1 open	Results
Efstathiou *et al.* (2008)	Identify health care users key areas of cancer care and services that needed to be developed or improved in Greece and prioritise them	Conventional 2 round	Purposive sample of 30 health care users (patients and carers) from two oncology and two general hospitals	• Knowledge and experience of living with cancer • Knowledge and experience of caring for a cancer patient • Using cancer services	To suggest the areas of cancer care and services, which needed developed or improved in Greece (Max of five suggestions)	123 statements generated collapsed into 27 themes
Ferguson *et al.* (2008)	Investigating consensus among physiotherapist in relation to the management of low back pain	Conventional 3 round	Purposive sample of 4 expert physiotherapists participated in Round 1 and 34 experts in subsequent rounds	• Working within one health board • Clinical grades (i.e. senior and clinical specialist) • Managed lower back pain on a regular basis	Based on a review of the literature 5 key questions were developed and agreed by 4 experts in focus groups. First round contained these 5 open questions	Not reported

Continued

Table 4.2 (*Continued*)

Author and year	Delphi focus	Delphi type and round number	Sample	Sample criteria	Round 1 open	Results
Whitehead (2005)	Gain consensus in relation to health promotion and health education constructs as they apply to nursing practice, education and policy	Conventional 2 rounds	Purposive sample of 62 international nursing experts	• Senior clinicians or academics servicing in nursing arenas • Involved in health promotion policy formation • Published works in health promotion disciplines • Possessed higher degree qualification	How do you view and define health promotion and health education?	134 statements generated collapsed into 13 categories
Beattie *et al.* (2004)	To gain consensus as to what a career pathway for nursing and midwifery should incorporate	Conventional 3 round	Purposive sample of 43 nurses and midwives identified via attendance at a consensus conference A further 13 were identified via expert contacts (snowball sampling)	• Registered nurse or midwife	If a new career pathway was introduced for nursing and midwifery in 2010, what would you consider to be its key features?	170 statements generated collapsed into 47 statements

Table 4.3 Example of closed Round 1

Author and year	Delphi focus	Delphi type and round number	Sample	Sample criteria	Round 1 open	Results
Malcolm *et al.* (2009)	To seek consensus amongst stakeholder groups (families, hospice staff/ volunteers and linked professionals) to rank research priorities for children's hospice care	Modified – 3 round Delphi	Stakeholders (621) (families *n* = 293; hospice staff/ volunteers n = 216 and professionals *n* = 112)	• Experiences of living with and/or caring for a child or young person with a limiting life condition and utilising or providing children's hospice services	Interviews with families (*n* = 5) linked professionals (*n* = 18) and focus groups with hospice staff and volunteers (*n* = 44) created 56 research topics categorised to 1 broad theme. Stakeholders (*n* = 621) asked to rate the importance of each topic and seek consensus on it being a future priority	44% response rate to Round 1
Jorm *et al.* (2008)	Achieve consensus on guidelines that could apply in a range of Asian countries to provide first aid to a person who is becoming psychotic	Modified – 3 round Delphi	Purposive sample of 59 mental health clinicians	• Graduate of the International Mental Health Leadership program	Web-administered questionnaire based on literature and reviewed by a working group. Respondents were asked to rate 211 statements on how important they believed it as a potential standard for mental health first aid for psychosis. Open questions also included	Items to be included *n* = 108 Items to be re-rated *n* = 41 New items added *n* = 8 Items to be excluded *n* = 62

Continued

Table 4.3 *(Continued)*

Author and year	Delphi focus	Delphi type and round number	Sample	Sample criteria	Round 1 open	Results
O'Brien *et al.* (2002)	Identify and agree upon the clinical indicators for mental health nursing standards of practice	Modified — 3 round Delphi	Purposive sample of 20 mental health nurses and 10 mental health consumers	• Expert nurses had to have a minimum of 3 years experience caring for mental health consumers • Expert consumer had to have 3 years of involvement as a consumer in mental health services	Questionnaire comprising of 91 clinical indicator statements, generated in focus groups of mental health nurses. On a 5-point Likert scale participants were asked to rate the importance of each clinical indicator. They were also asked to suggest additional indicators they felt were pivotal	An additional 21 clinical indicators were identified

Wellar (2008) found that a small panel size of ten provided a diversity of expert opinion, while Jones and Twiss (1978) recommended 10–50 participants whereas Wild and Torgersen (2000b) suggested a panel size of 300–500 to provide representative information.

Cantrill *et al.* (1996) have noted that virtually any panel size have been utilised in health applications, ranging in the number of participants from 4 to 3000. Although Akins *et al.* (2005) reported that most published Delphi sample sizes consist of 10 to 100 experts; studies with less than 10 participants have also been reported. For example, Malone *et al.* (2005) explored drug interactions in ambulatory pharmacy settings with five experts while Strasser *et al.* (2005) explored competence training for primary care nurses with six experts.

However, the Delphi technique does not advocate the inclusion of a random sample of experts who are representative (Goodman, 1987) essentially, the number of participants is dependent upon the topic under investigation, the relevant perspectives required, complexity of the problem, design selected, representation, resources available and range of expertise required (Whitman, 1990; Loo, 2002; Powell, 2003; de Villiers *et al.*, 2005; Turoff, 2006). It is recommended that if the sample is homogeneous, then a smaller sample size, such as 10–15 participants (Delbecq *et al.*, 1975; Skulmoski *et al.*, 2007) may be sufficient, as you could infer that the results are generalisable and representative to the larger population. In contrast, if the sample is heterogeneous more subjects may be required; however, this may require additional resources to administer and analyse the volume of resulting data.

Response rate and attrition

No specific guidelines exist for an acceptable response rate for Delphi studies. A review of Delphi literature reveals variations in response rates from 8% (Cooney *et al.*, 1995) to 100% (Pilon *et al.*, 1995; McKenna *et al.*, 2003; Owens *et al.*, 2008). A number of authors (Bork, 1993; Walker & Selfe, 1996; Sumsion, 1998) recommend a 70% response rate is necessary for each round to maintain rigor. However, achieving this requires considerable effort.

Attrition can occur in any type of research study, however, as the Delphi has several rounds there is a higher potential for experts to withdraw from the study due to fatigue, distractions between rounds or disillusionment with the process (Donohoe & Needham, 2008). Worthen and Saunders (1987) believe that after the third round attrition is most likely to occur. However, attrition can occur at any stage, for example at Round 1 or as both Farrel and Scherer (1983) and McKenna (1994a) suggested high dropout rates characterise the final rounds of most Delphi's. For example, Alexandrov *et al.* (1996) reported a dropout rate of 28% between investigator selection and their first response, while Day and Bobeva (2005) experienced a 40% dropout rate after Round 1. A notable study was undertaken by Mayaka and King (2002), who had to confine their Delphi study to one round due to unwillingness of panellists to participate in subsequent rounds.

Evans (1997) suggested that large Delphi panels have a higher attrition rate, while panels with an initially small pool of responses may experience low or non-existent dropout rates. In both cases, bias may enter into the study due to a high attrition rate with a larger sample and a potentially unrepresentative small sample at the study's inception. Dropout can lead to a response bias if the attrition rate is substantial; therefore, the researcher must try to reduce this occurrence. A number of strategies can be used to aid the inclusion and commitment from panel members; these include the following:

- At the outset provide prospective panel members with a clear explanation of the Delphi process, explaining that their commitment to participate would involve several rounds of questionnaires and feedback extending over a period of months (Needham & De Loe, 1990; Loo, 2002).
- Obtain participants written consent and/or intention to commit to Delphi rounds (Rudy, 1996). (See Chapter 8 for an example of a consent form)
- Depending upon resources available, some authors (Mitchell, 1991; McKenna, 1994a) advocated the use of face-to-face interviews to develop rapport, respond to initial questions and to add a 'personal touch'.
- Ongoing (e-mail, phone and written) communication, incentives and continual reminders, can be used throughout the research process to recruit and retain panel members (Sandrey & Bulger, 2008).
- Quick turnaround times in data collection can enhance enthusiasm and reduce dropouts (Gordon, 1994).
- Conduct the study based around respondents' work and holiday schedules (Franklin & Hart, 2007), creating a comprehensive panel management plan (Moeller & Shafer, 1994; Andronovich, 1995; Briedenhann & Butts, 2006).
- Consider limiting the number of rounds to two or three to reduce panel fatigue occurring (Linstone & Turoff, 1975).
- Assess panel stability throughout the process with a quality control measure based on predetermined panel composition preferences and criteria (Garrod & Fyall, 2005).
- More importantly, a researcher should aim to communicate the ongoing importance of each individual panel member's contribution to the research process (Sandrey & Bulger, 2008) and the impact his/her involvement will have on the research outcome.

Interacting with Delphi participants can be time-consuming; however, it can help mediate additional problems, increase understanding of the approach and encourage participation. Therefore, when using a Delphi researchers can never rest on their laurels of initially recruiting panel members, considerable effort needs to be made at very round to ensure dropouts do not occur.

Deciding on nature and delivery of the first round

As the Delphi method does not require participants to meet face to face, there is little opportunity to ensure that the participants fully comprehend the purpose of the study (Murray & Hammons, 1995); therefore, careful consideration needs to be given to the development of Round 1. Franklin and Hart (2007) warned that developing the first round of a Delphi can be difficult. Essentially, there are two options available for researchers to design the first round of a Delphi.

The first reflects the traditional approach, which begins with an open qualitative round in the form of an open-ended question. Panel members can be asked to provide one word, phrase, sentence or paragraph as a response (Cochran, 1983). In essence, this approach reflects a brainstorming session (Murry & Hammons, 1995) and serves as the foundation for soliciting information on the topic area and upon which the Delphi is based. Careful consideration, however, must be given to avoid vague questions which can result in ambiguous responses (Sackman, 1975; Couper, 1984) and, therefore, limit the reliability and validity of the data. To ensure clarity a pilot test of Round 1 is recommended (Miller, 2001). This open approach ensures that panel members have the opportunity to provide the intricacies of an issue and space to express themselves in their own words. However, this relies on respondents making the effort to list the complexity of the issue and quite often results in large amounts of raw data to analyse. For example, Cochran (1983) suggests about 100 statements can be generated from Round 1. Numerous examples of an opening first round are cited in the literature (see Table 4.2).

The second approach requires the researcher to identify those issues of high pertinence. Therefore, the panel is given pre-selected issues upon which to make a judgement, these can be developed upon a review of the literature, interviews, focus groups or other forms of consultation with key stakeholders (Lang, 1994; Eggers & Jones, 1998; Keeney et al., 2006). This approach is often referred to as a 'modified' Delphi as it dispenses with the traditional open-ended format. Table 4.3 outlines some of the varying approaches adopted in the literature. This approach orientates panellists and ensures that everyone starts from a common base and does lend itself easier to statistical analysis and interpretation. However, this tactic does create its own drawbacks, for example the response choices must be known in advance; it does not provide the respondent with an opportunity to supply answers which may not 'fit' into the range of options supplied (Denscombe, 2003), which could bias responses.

Deciding on the nature of the first round is a significant decision which needs to be considered early in the research design phase. Regardless of which approach adopted, it should always be piloted.

Gaining names and addresses

In any type of research, gaining the contact details of respondents can be challenging; however, the approach adopted is heavily dependent upon the sampling approach selected. For example, many sampling frames may already contain names and addresses, yet exigencies of carrying out research in reality can mean that such lists may be impossible to obtain, be out of date or otherwise incorrect. A number of approaches have been adopted to facilitate access to panel members' details, for example Moreno-Casbas et al. (2001) used conference and discussion lists to identify some panel members, Annells et al. (2005) utilised employment lists, while Klimenko and Julliard (2007) identified their sample via literature and Internet searches and by seeking the opinion of representatives of specific areas of health care.

As recommended by Vernon (2009) once participants have been identified it is usual to invite them to take part before commencing with Round 1 of the Delphi. When accessing panellists details a number of issues should be considered including gatekeepers, ethics and researchers negotiating and interpersonal skills (Pole & Lampard, 2002). Firstly, the role of the gatekeeper is vital in many research studies, as he/she may have the power to influence access to research setting and participants. Researchers, therefore, need to identify who holds this position and to develop strong links with this person to enhance their, and consequently the panellists' commitment to the study. Secondly, gaining access to a research setting and the names of potential study members may be dependent on formal ethics committee approval. Although this can be time-consuming and does in no way guarantee members will participate, it can reassure wary respondents and assurances of anonymity and confidentiality may also enhance responses. Finally, the researcher's personality and interpersonal skills can play an important role at this stage (Burgess, 1984). Pole and Lampard (2002) claim that the status and visible characteristics of the researcher may influence access to some contexts a fact that can be applied to most research settings. For example, a researcher having links with or a role within the research setting may be advantageous in helping to overcome initial barriers and establishing rapport with gatekeepers.

Deciding on a 'return by' date

Delbecq et al. (1975) recommended that Delphi panellists be given 2 weeks to respond to each round. Less than one week may not allow the participant the time to complete the round, while over 2 weeks may result it becoming a low priority and never being completed. The completion of a round should take up to 30 minutes (Mitchell, 1991); however, this is dependent on the complexity of the topic under investigation and the size of the panel.

Administration

Given the methodological complexity of a Delphi, a researcher has numerous administrative responsibilities and duties to undertake, such as, sending an initial letter of invitation, designing the questionnaire, cover letter, developing coding systems to track respondents, creating file systems for responses and creating and maintaining mailing databases (See Chapter 8).

Invitation to participate

Once a perspective panellist has been identified, he or she may be contacted to gain initial consent to take part in the study. Contact can be via phone or written communication or both, for example a phone call followed by an invitation letter. Initial contact may also provide the opportunity for snowballing to occur that is asking the potential participant if they can nominate someone else for the study. Cochran (1983) suggested that this invitation should explain what the study is about, provides information about the Delphi method, explains the commitment sought and formally asks the individual to become a member of the panel. Initial contact should also explain how the panellists have been identified and why they are being approached. Figure 4.1 outlines an example of a letter of invitation used in a conventional Delphi study.

Initial invitations can also offer and gain confirmation of the most suitable choice of communication methods for each panellist, such as e-mail, written or online to participants. Researchers can sometimes find multi-mode communication methods may be adopted in one single Delphi study, to cater to panellists who prefer e-mail and those who prefer pen and pencil responses. Invitation letters are often accompanied by more extensive detailed instructions (including a participant information sheet, consent form and a stamped addressed envelope, see Chapter 8 for examples).

A number of studies have formally invited panel members to take part in the study before the first round is disseminated (see Kilroy & Driscoll, 2006; Hung *et al.*, 2008; Watson, 2008). Gaining initial commitment of the panel and providing information on how the study will be implemented may help to ensure that the respondents feel sufficient ownership of the study.

Once participation has been confirmed, this is followed up with an initial questionnaire mailing within 1–2 weeks.

Dear Sir/ Madam,

Re: ≪insert study title≫

The ≪insert organisation≫ have been commissioned by the ⌐insert funder name⌐ to identify research priorities for the Therapy Professions as perceived by professionals working in clinical areas, academics working in higher education institutions and key stakeholders, such as voluntary sector, statutory bodies and service users. The Therapy professions (chiropody/podiatry, dietetics, occupational therapy, orthoptics, physiotherapy and speech and language therapy) constitute a growing proportion of the public health care workforce, playing a significant role in the provision of health care. There is little research to date which has examined the research priorities of the Therapy professions. This research will, therefore, ensure a more focused, coherent and coordinated approach to guide future therapy research and to ensure that investment ensures optimal delivery of services at a systems and individual level.

The study has inclusion criteria which we think you might meet. This inclusion criteria for your profession is as follows:

- Must have 3 years post-qualification experience in the clinical area
- Must be currently employed in a clinical area
- Willing to participate

If you do meet the inclusion criteria and would be willing to participate in the study, we would be very grateful if you could complete the enclosed consent form and return it in the stamped addressed envelope provided before ≪insert return date≫.

This research will be carried out using the Delphi technique consisting of 3 questionnaires (known as rounds) aiming to achieve consensus. With your permission the questionnaires will be posted or e-mailed to you. After receipt of the enclosed consent form, you will shortly receive the first questionnaire. Simple and specific instructions will be provided for each questionnaire.

The amount of time necessary for completion of each questionnaire (or rounds) will vary with each panellist, but should range from approximately 15–30 minutes for Round 1, 10–20 minutes for Round 2, and 20–30 minutes for Round 3. There are no right or wrong answers to the questions. This study is seeking your expert opinion. We think you will find the process interesting and results will be made available at you at the conclusion of this study.

It is important that you understand that your participation in this study is entirely voluntary. If you do not wish to take part in this study it will not affect your employment or service provided. In addition, any information that you provide will be confidential and when the results of the study are reported, you will not be identifiable in the findings. Your name will not be recorded on any rounds; instead, you will be allocated a unique code that can only be identifiable to the researcher. You will remain anonymous to the other participants (or experts) throughout this Delphi study and only the researchers will be able to identify your specific answers. Return of completed Delphi rounds implies consent to participate.

We sincerely hope you will agree to participate. If you have any questions please, e-mail ≪researcher's e-mail address≫ or call ≪researcher's telephone number≫.

Thank you for your time and any help you may be able to offer to this study.

Yours sincerely

≪insert name, tile and organisation≫

Figure 4.1   Example of Letter of Invitation

Explicit cover letter outlining the working of the Delphi

A cover letter is vital for any Delphi study especially as participants may be unfamiliar with the technique. Evidence suggests cover letters can help persuade recipients to participate by stressing the importance of their involvement (Zeinio, 1980; Loo, 2002) and has been effective in numerous Delphi projects (Whitman, 1990). Consideration should also be given towards personalising correspondence including cover letters to panellists.

The initial cover letter, accompanied with Round 1, needs to detail specific information, for example:

- Brief outline of the project
- Emphasise its importance and why it is of benefit to the individual
- Explain the Delphi process that is the anticipated number of rounds, time commitment, and the format for responses
- Provide assurances of confidentiality
- If necessary explain why identification numbers are being used
- Provide contact details of the researcher if questions should arise
- Thank the participant for their assistance
- Signature including the job title and position of the sender

(*Source*: Dillman, 1978; Gordon, 1994)

A cover letter is also accompanied by more extensive detailed instructions (including a demographic sheet (see Figure 4.2) and a stamped addressed envelope). Instructions should be developed and sent with each individual round. Figures 4.3 and 4.4 outline an example of a Round 1 cover letter and instructions to panellists. Two to three days after Round 1 has been disseminated the researcher should contact each panellist to ensure that materials have been received, and to answer any initial queries (Novakowski & Wellar, 2008). Any issues identified at this initial stage need to be responded to promptly and consistently. Adopting this approach will help build upon the researcher–panellist relationship and potentially encourage response rates.

Design of questionnaire

Similar to developing any survey, the design of a Round 1 questionnaire needs careful consideration. Once you have established what information is required, the panel members to target and the nature of the first round (open or closed) you then need to draft Round 1, considering content, format, structure and layout. Loo (2002) believes that developing the questionnaire for Round 1 is similar to any survey being mindful of questionnaire design good practice, for example the length of the questionnaire should be kept short to enhance response rates (Edwards *et al.*, 2002), ensure wording is unambiguous and provide sufficient room for responses.

Current employment

Name: _____

Present job title: _____

Department: _____

Employing organisation: _____

Background details *(please tick)*

Are you…	**Male**	☐	**Female**	☐
What age are you?	18–24	☐	45–54	☐
	25–34	☐	55–65	☐
	35–44	☐	Over 65	☐

If applicable, please list your qualifications

_____

_____

If applicable, please indicate how many years experience since qualifying

_____

_____

If applicable, do you work in the health service or in private practice?

Health service ☐   Private practice ☐

Please tick, which therapies professions you work in:

Chiropody/podiatry	☐	Orthoptics	☐
Dietetics	☐	Physiotherapy	☐
Occupational therapy	☐	Speech and language therapy	☐
None of the above	☐	*(Please state………………..)*	

Thank you for taking the time to complete this first round questionnaire.
Please return the questionnaire in the stamped addressed envelope enclosed by
insert return date.

Figure 4.2   Demographics sheet

Dear ≪insert recipient name≫,

Re: A study to identify research priorities for the therapy professions

Thank you for returning your consent form indicating that you meet the inclusion criteria for this study and that you are willing to participate.

You will find enclosed with this letter an instruction sheet and the first round Delphi questionnaire. The aim of this study is to come to agreement on the research priorities for the therapies at present.

Please read the instructions carefully and complete the Delphi questionnaire as fully as you can. It is also important that you complete the demographics sheet at the end of the questionnaire as this will enable the research team to provide you with feedback throughout the process. Return of completed Delphi round implies consent to participate.

If you could return the questionnaire in the enclosed stamped addressed envelope by ≪insert return date≫ we would be most grateful. If you wish to discuss any aspect of this further, please contact ≪insert researcher's details≫.

Thank you for agreeing to participate in this study.

Yours sincerely,

≪insert title, name and organisation≫

Figure 4.3   Example of a Round 1 Delphi cover letter

The next step is to identify and develop the actual question(s) which you need to ask, the nature of which is dependent upon the aims and objectives of the study. There are general principles to abide by to minimise respondent misunderstanding or response bias, for example keep the question short, keep the vocabulary simple, avoid double-barrelled questions and hypothetical questions and be aware of leading questions (Siniscalco & Auriat, 2005). In addition, emotive words or phases should not be used (Rowe & Wright, 2001). Figure 4.5 provides an illustration of a Round 1 used in a Delphi study. Although not included in the example outlined, a researcher may wish to ask panellists, especially if using

Instructions on how to complete Delphi Round 1

The first round of this Delphi will ask you a question – 'What are the research priorities for your profession at present?'

There are ten spaces for you to detail your answers. You can complete as many or as few of these spaces as you wish. Please be as detailed in your response as possible.

Please complete the demographics sheet at the end of the questionnaire. It is important that the researcher can identify your responses as the Delphi process has individual feedback to every panel member built into the process.

Once you have completed the questionnaire, please return it to the researcher in the enclosed stamped addressed envelope by ≪return date≫.

Figure 4.4   Instructions to Delphi Round 1

Identification of research priorities for the therapies professions

Delphi Round 1

Please list your answers to the following question. You can list as many answer as you wish and they do not have to be in any particular order.

Question: What are the current research priorities for your profession?

_____

_____

_____

_____

_____

_____

_____

_____

_____

_____

_____

_____

Figure 4.5   Example of Delphi Round 1

a heterogeneous sample, to rate their confidence in their answers and/or provide a 'no judgement' option for those who do not have an opinion (Turoff, 2006).

Whilst Moore (1987) viewed pilot testing as being optional, for others it is a crucial element of a good Delphi research design (Mitchell, 1991; Gordon, 1994; Novakowski & Wellar, 2008). Pilot testing refers to undertaking a trial run using the full-blown draft Delphi survey and testing in on a small sample panel (Novakowski & Wellar, 2008). For example, Mohorjy and Aburizaiza (1997) pre-tested their Delphi questionnaire by sending a random mailing to 10% of their expert panel. Whilst this initially can seem as extra work the value in identifying wording ambiguities (Turoff, 1975), improving administration systems (Jillson, 1975a) and providing information regarding their reliability and validity (Jairath & Weinstein, 1994) is worth the effort. With most research you get only one opportunity to collect the data; therefore, as van Teijlingen and Hundley (2001) suggested a pilot study may provide you an advanced warning about where the main study could fail.

Administration systems

In a Delphi study, the development and administration of questionnaires are interconnected (Ludwing, 1997). This entails three main features: firstly, developing coding systems to track respondents, creating file systems to record responses generating and maintaining mailing databases. Before dissemination all panel members should be assigned a code (or ID number), which should be clearly recorded on the initial and subsequent rounds. By doing so, you will be able to link responses, follow up nonresponses and remove names from their questionnaires to ensure confidentiality. The next step is to develop a file system which will contain the panellist's unique ID number and his/her responses to each round. This is a vital aspect for the Delphi process as in subsequent rounds panellists are fed back individual as well as group responses. A researcher should also create a filing system (linked again with the ID) to record if a reminder has been sent and if so what type and to detail all other relevant correspondence. Finally, a master list of the ID numbers and corresponding names should be developed. This can be much more than a simple list of names and address, this can also contain panellists preferred mode of contact (i.e. e-mail or phone), times when they will be available or other identifying makers.

The development of such system may seem straightforward but they are time-consuming to create and to maintain. Administrative errors can impede the progress of any research; to ensure the effective progression of a Delphi study it needs to be well planned and administration systems subject to pilot-testing.

Mailing

Traditionally, a Delphi has been conducted using postal mail; however, with advancement of technology, the option of e-mail and web-based Delphi projects opens new possibilities, which can speed up the time line from months to a few weeks (Loo, 2002; Donohoe & Needham, 2008). When using the traditional postal service, consideration needs to be given towards stationary required and cost factors. Traditionally, in Round 1 of a conventional Delphi panellists are mailed a cover letter, Round 1 questionnaire with instructions for completion, and a self-addressed return envelope. As a researcher you may also want to use this opportunity to include a demographic questionnaire to provide data on the qualifications, experience, job description and demographics of your sample.

Maximising response rate

Given the Delphi process, considerable effort must be made to ensure participants stay motivated and committed to several rounds. The use of reminders is endorsed in general texts for surveys (Edwards *et al.*, 2002) and Delphi's are no different. Dillman's (1978) Total Design Method advocates three follow-up contacts. The first is a postcard, normally sent 1 week after the round has been sent, this is sent to all panel members thanking those who have returned the questionnaire and reminding those who have not yet done so, that there is still time to do so. In case the respondent mislays the original questionnaire, the second reminder is a reminder letter and a replacement questionnaire sent to non-respondents 3 weeks after the initial questionnaire. Finally, a letter and replacement questionnaire is sent to non-respondents, which Dillman (1978) suggests should be sent by recorded mail.

There are also a number of other strategies a researcher can adopt to enhance response rates; these include the following:

- Clearly informing respondents from the outset what the study goal is, why they are being involved, who will see the results and how the results will be used. Establishing and reminding panellists at every round the benefits of the results, how they may be put into action or impact upon practice should be specified.
- Precautions taken to protect the anonymity and confidentiality of panellists' responses should be clearly communicated. If assurances are made that individual answers will not be linked to individual responses in any way, panellists may feel more likely to respond and provide truthful answers. This is discussed further in Chapter 8. Some researchers (Rauch, 1979) have used quasi-anonymity to enhance response rates. The fact that respondents may know that they are

involved in a Delphi study; Rauch (1979) postulated that this should have the effect of motivating the panellists to participate.

- While obvious the maintenance of good administration systems to ensure identification of respondents and non-respondents is required.
- Establish a deadline for returns for each Delphi round and inform participants in all forms of communications this date. A timeframe of 7–10 days should be available.
- Insert clear instructions on how long it will take to complete each round and whom to contact if a question arises.
- The value of the personal touch cannot be underestimated in a Delphi study. Paying individual attention to panel members will help to develop solid working relationships which Novakowski and Wellar (2008) suggest can result in faster responses. Building relationships and being able to directly speak to panellists on the phone can also help enhance response rates. Such contact can also help to answer queries about the Delphi process.
- Finally, keep it brief, panellists are normally busy people; therefore, their time is precious, taking part in a Delphi study may not be their primary concern, unlike the researcher.

Content analysis

There is no standard approach used to analyse data from Delphi rounds. Jairath and Weinstein (1994) claimed that analysis is affected by the purpose of the study, structure of rounds, types of questions (closed or open-ended) and the number of respondents. Normally, when an open-ended question is employed in the first round, a vast number of interrelated items may be produced. For example, in Table 4.2 (Efstathiou *et al.*, 2008) open Round 1 resulted in 123 statements being identified which reduced to 27 themes.

In order to condense the data for Round 2, content analysis to identify major themes may be sufficient (Powell, 2003). This requires similar items to be combined or collapsed with decisions to be made on items occurring infrequently on whether they should be included or omitted. A researcher has a big task to ensure that the resulting list is kept manageable (Whitman, 1990); however, as this process does not provide the opportunity to interact with participants to elaborate their views or explain their rationale behind their response, this process has the potential to introduce researcher bias (Goodman, 1987; Walker & Selfe, 1996; Sumsion, 1998).

Content analysis can be undertaken manually or by software packages. Manually analysing qualitative data is time-consuming as it requires reading and re-reading of responses, developing a process of coding, categorising and conceptualising the responses. There are a number of sources of different frameworks to help in undertaking content analysis (see, for example Burnard, 1991; Miles & Huberman, 1994). Qualitative research software (e.g., NUD*IST) essentially enables qualitative data to be organised and cross-referenced easily. While it also encourages consistent coding and categorisation of the data, they are not a short-cut as it can take time to develop proficiency in their use and the process of developing codes and categories still has to be made (Lathlean, 2005).

As with any research, methodological rigor needs to be considered, this is critical for qualitative (Sandleowski, 1986) and quantitative research (Creswell, 1994). Issues relating to trustworthiness for qualitative open round and reliability and validity for subsequent quantitative rounds must also be considered (Polit *et al.*, 2001)

Process

The success of a Delphi lies within its planning. With no scientific guidance, interpretative freedom and flexibility with the technique exist; nevertheless, a researcher should follow a set of general rules to instil confidence in the research results (Moeller & Shafer, 1994; Briedenhann & Butts, 2006). Table 4.4 summarises some of the key steps, for example define and state the level of consensus to be applied, provide a clear rationale for the use of the Delphi, the sample to be identified and the nature of the first round.

Table 4.4 Plan for getting started

Step 1	Literature review Establish the need for the research Review and confirm the Delphi is the most appropriate method Review availability of resources
Step 2	Identify and define the level of consensus to be applied
Step 3	Identification of potential target population Agree on method of selection of expert panel Review and agree sample size Gain the names and address of potential expert panel Develop strategies to enhance response rates Develop administration procedures
Step 4	Decide on the nature of the first round Decide on a return date
Step 5	Draft Round 1 documentation, letter of invitation and Round 1 pack (including cover letter, Round 1 questionnaire, instructions and stamped addressed envelope)
Step 6	Select Delphi members Select trial run candidates Pilot test Round 1 pack and administration systems and review where necessary
Step 7	Distribution of Round 1

Give careful consideration to the skills available, the time required to develop and maintain administration systems. Undertaking some of these initial steps may help to avoid or minimise dilemmas faced in the field later.

Key learning points

- Effective planning underpins the success of any Delphi study.
- Initial considerations should focus on the suitability of the method, analysis of resources available and consideration of the consensus level to be applied.
- Identifying, targeting, selecting, recruiting and maintaining a Delphi's expert panel requires intense effort.
- The first round of a Delphi can be an open qualitative round to solicit information or closed consisting of pre-selected issues upon which panellists make a judgement.
- Experts contact details can be obtained from a number of sources, that is, conference lists, literature review or employment lists. The importance of gatekeepers, ethics and researchers negotiating and interpersonal skills should not be underestimated.
- A researcher has numerous administrative responsibilities, such as sending an initial letter of invitation, designing the questionnaire, cover letter, developing coding systems creating and maintaining file and mailing databases.
- Once a perspective panellist has been identified, an invitation (verbal followed by written communication) should be issued.
- Designing and developing the Delphi questions is dependent upon the aims and objectives of the study.
- The decision on which method of delivery to adopt (i.e. postal, e-mail or both) needs to reflect the needs and skills of the expert panel.
- In Round 1, each participant should be sent an explicit cover letter, instructions, demographic questionnaire (optimal) and the Delphi.
- Strategies to maximise response rates throughout the Delphi process should be adopted.
- Normally open-ended questions are subject to content analysis.
- Undertaking a pilot study may provide you an advanced warning about where the main study could fail.

Recommended further reading

Geist, M. (2009) Using the Delphi method to engage stakeholders: a comparison of two studies. *Evaluation and Program Planning* 23(2), 147–154.

Green, B., Jones, M., Hughes, D. & Williams A. (1999) Applying the Delphi technique in a study of GPs information requirements. *Health and Social Care in the Community* 7(3) 198–205.

Keeney, S., Hasson, F. & McKenna, H.P. (2006) Consulting the oracle: ten lessons from using the Delphi technique in nursing research. *Journal of Advanced Nursing* 53(2), 205–212.

5 Conducting the Research Using the Delphi Technique

Introduction

As has been referred to in the previous chapters, the Delphi technique employs a number of rounds in which questionnaires are sent out until consensus is reached (Beretta, 1996; Green *et al.*, 1999). In each round, a summary of the results of the previous round is included and evaluated by the expert panel members. McKenna (1994a) implied that this process facilitates the 'systematic emergence of a concurrence of judgement/opinion' (p. 1222). As Chapter 4 has shown, the number of rounds depends upon the time available and whether the Delphi has started with one broad question or with a list of questions or events. This process raises the question of how many rounds it takes to reach consensus. The classical original Delphi used four rounds (Young & Hogben, 1978). However, as has been illustrated in the previous chapters, this has been modified by many authors to suit individual research aims and, in some cases, it has been shortened to two or three rounds (Beech, 1997). It is also difficult to retain a high response rate within a 'Delphi' that has many rounds. The topic needs to be of great interest to the panel members or they need to be rewarded in other ways. This chapter sets out the process of the Delphi from Round 1 to the end of the process.

First round

Classical Delphi

Round 1 of the classical Delphi starts with an open-ended set of questions, thus allowing panel members freedom in their responses. The number of items generated can be extremely large, especially if the researcher opts for an inclusive approach. Proctor and Hunt (1994) stated that the Delphi process can produce 'large and unwieldy amounts of information particularly if the researcher adopts a qualitative stance towards the data and is

The Delphi Technique in Nursing and Health Research, First Edition, © S. Keeney, F. Hasson and H. McKenna   Published 2011 by Blackwell Publishing Ltd.

reluctant to collapse categories' (p. 1004). Unfortunately, this tendency to include all panel members' Round 1 views can create very lengthy second-round questionnaires. Being all-inclusive can put panel members off participating and it can become very difficult to sustain the experts' interest in the study (Green *et al.*, 1999). A further critique concerns the view that if questions are not well phrased and definitive, the reliability and validity of data may be threatened.

Traditionally, Round 1 is used to generate ideas and the panel members are asked for their responses to or comments about an issue. There is now some support for revising the approach and providing pre-existing information for ranking or response. However, it must be recognised that this approach could bias the responses or limit the available options. Nonetheless, a clear advantage to commencing the process in this way is that it could be more efficient in a technique that has the potential to be very time-consuming (Jenkins & Smith, 1994).

Therefore, Round 1 of the classical Delphi is a qualitative round. The expert panel will have been recruited as discussed in Chapter 4. Each member will have received a detailed description of the study and a Participant Information Sheet. They will also have signed a consent form which will be held by the researcher (see Chapter 8 for information on participant information sheets and consent forms).

With the Round 1 questionnaire, the researcher should send an information pack to each panel member which should include a cover letter and instructions on how to complete the Round 1 questionnaire. An example of the type of cover letter that should be used is illustrated from a study undertaken by the authors into research priorities for the therapies professions. An example of the type of instructions that should be included is also set out from the same study. Chapter 4 also sets out the design of the first round questionnaire. In this example, the questionnaire was also designed to collect demographic information from the expert panel, such as age, gender, years experience, qualifications and which of the therapies professions that they work in. The reason for this was to be able to describe the sample in those terms. However, this is not essential for a Delphi study and, indeed, many studies will not deem it necessary to collect this information.

Modified Delphi

Obviously, in a modified Delphi, the open ended round of a classical Delphi does not take place. The three main modifications made to replace this Round 1 are as follows:

1. Developing statements from the existing literature in the field
2. Undertaking focus groups
3. Undertaking one-to-one interviews

Any of these modifications require content analysis of the results following a similar process as the Round 1 results from an open-ended first round. An appropriate content analysis framework should be used, such as Burnard (1991) or any of the frameworks discussed in Chapter 4.

Return of first round

The expert panel should be asked to return the Round 1 questionnaire in the stamped addressed envelope (SAE) to the research team. The SAE should be provided by the researcher with the Round 1 questionnaire. A return date should be given for return. Reminders are very important between the Delphi rounds (Edwards *et al.*, 2002). One week before the return date a set of reminders should be sent to those members of the expert panel who have not yet returned the questionnaire. This can be done by post or e-mail, usually in whichever manner the questionnaire has been sent initially. A further reminder should be sent one week after the return date. Some Delphi researchers also advocate telephoning those members of the expert panel to speak with them about their participation in the study (Sandrey & Bulger, 2008). However, this could be considered coercion by the researcher to take part in the study and should be considered carefully before using this method. Chapter 4 outlines the use of Dillman's (1978) Total Design Method to aid follow-up of questionnaires.

Consideration of sample size and number of items generated

Careful consideration should be given to the number of items or priorities that a Delphi researcher allows each expert panel member to specify while using the classical Delphi and a qualitative (open) first round. The prime concern here is that the more items the researcher allows an expert panel member to specify, the more items you will have to content analyse and, more important, return to the expert panel in the next round. Response rate has to be balanced with quantity and breadth of the study in this regard. There is no point in having a wide and all-encompassing study if the response rate is 10%. However, at the other extreme, it would not be useful to have a study with 100% response rate with only a handful of statements for the panel to consider. On balance, when using a qualitative first round it is prudent to allow an expert panel to identify a minimum five items/priorities and a maximum of ten items/priorities. This should safeguard against an unmanageable number of items for the second round and should ensure a reasonable to good response rate. The response rate can be enhanced in other ways including building up a good relationship with your panel and in the selection of the panel in the first instance.

See Chapters 1 and 4 for more information on response rates in Delphi studies.

Bootstrapping

Bootstrapping is a general purpose approach to statistical inference which falls within a broader definition of re-sampling methods. It is the practice of estimating properties of an estimator (such as its variance) by measuring those properties when sampling from an approximating distribution. One standard choice for an approximating distribution is the empirical distribution of the observed data. In the case where a set of observations can be assumed to be from an independent and identically distributed population, this can be implemented by constructing a number of re-samples of the observed dataset (and of equal size to the observed dataset), each of which is obtained by random sampling within replacement from the original dataset.

The use of bootstrapping within the Delphi technique was demonstrated by Akins *et al.* (2005) in a study with 23 experts in health care quality and patient safety. The authors acknowledged that there is no clear consensus on how many experts should participate in Delphi rounds to ensure stability of responses. The responses from the 23 experts constituted one sample in the study were augmented via bootstrapping to obtain computer-generated sample for much larger panels of 1000 and 2000 participants using re-sampling iterations. Findings from the study show that the responses from a small number of experts ($n = 23$) in a focused area of knowledge are stable in the light of augmented sampling.

Content analysis

Round 1 of the classical Delphi should be content analysed in order to group statements generated by the expert panel into similar areas. Any type of content analysis framework can be used for this but in this regard due to the nature of the data and the required analysis a simple approach to content analysing usually works well. An approach, such as Burnard (1991), would give a useful framework for analysis as outlined in Table 5.1. In many respects, the aim of this exercise is to group all similar statements into areas and then examine each area for statements that are either exactly the same and can be collapsed into one statement or which are similar. If statements are similar, a decision should be made on whether they can be collapsed into one statement without changing the meaning or whether they are sufficiently different to warrant returning them as different statements in Round 2 of the Delphi. Again, consideration should be given to the numbers of statements included in Round

Table 5.1   Outline of Burnard's (1991) method of content analysis: 14 stage process

1. Make notes memos post interview
2. Read transcripts and note general themes
3. Note as many headings as required
4. Categories are grouped together
5. Remove repetitive headings
6. Two researchers independently generate categories from data
7. Transcripts re-read alongside list of categories
8. Each transcript worked through and coded
9. Coded sections cut and collapsed together
10. All collapsed sections organised under headings
11. Some participants asked to check
12. All sections filed for write up
13. Access to original transcripts – write up
14. Use of literature (separate or integrate)

Source: Adapted from Burnard (1991).

2 in relation to the response rate. The longer the Round 2 questionnaire, the less likely expert panel members will be to fill it in which is always a consideration with any type of survey research.

Subsequent rounds

Rounds 2–4 take the form of structured questionnaires incorporating feedback to each panel member. These rounds are analysed and re-circulated and it has been shown that this process encourages panel members to become more involved and motivated to participate (Walker & Selfe, 1996). In this way, the Delphi allows efficient and rapid collection of expert opinions, while the feedback is controlled (Buck *et al.*, 1993). The ability of the Delphi to involve and motivate panel members means that they can be involved actively in the development of the instrument: this leads to perceptions of ownership and acceptance of the findings (McKenna, 1994a). The active involvement of staff in the identification of their own development needs is crucial for the success of any development program (Shepard, 1995). This can be viewed as an incentive and major advantage in using this technique.

The Delphi often collects qualitative and quantitative data yet little guidance exists in relation to the balance of data collected and how to manage the data generated (Green *et al.*, 1999). The lack of guidance leads to a variety of approaches and can result in different Delphi studies interpreting and reporting in different ways: this could affect the integrity of the method.

As discussed previously, the Delphi technique might encounter problems due to a decline in response rate because, in order to achieve consensus, it is important that those panel members who have agreed to participate stay involved until the process is completed (Buck *et al.*, 1993). However, poor response rates are a characterisation of the final round of the Delphi. This could be why many researchers are now stopping at two or three rounds rather than the originally recommended four rounds. McKenna (1994b), however, found that using face-to-face interviews in the first round increases the return rates of postal questionnaires in the second, concluding that panel members appeared to appreciate the 'personal touch'.

Round 2

Round 2 of a classical Delphi questionnaire should be designed using the generated items from Round 1. It is sometime useful if Round 2 is a lengthy questionnaire to group statements into specific areas so that panel members can work through each area separately. Panel members should be sent a cover letter, a set of instructions for Round 2, the Round 2 questionnaire and an SAE. Within the Round 2 Delphi questionnaire, research priorities or items should be listed and expert panel members should be asked to rate each of the priorities or items on an appropriate scale. This could be a seven-point Likert scale from 'very important' to 'unimportant' or a five point scale from 'strongly agree to strongly disagree'. They should be asked to return the completed questionnaire within the given time period using the enclosed SAE. A master code should link each expert panel members' responses to each round. This list of master codes should be known only to the researcher. As with Round 1, follow-up reminders should be sent to expert panel members as necessary. As Round 2 can be a time when many expert panel members can drop out, every effort should be made at this stage to maintain the expert panel members' interest in the study (Linstone & Turoff, 1975; Gordon, 1994; Loo, 2002; Sandrey & Bulger, 2008).

Cover letter explaining Round 2

Round 2 of the Delphi technique should be sent to the expert panel with a clear cover letter and instructions on how to complete the Round 2 questionnaire. This is especially important in the classical Delphi as this round will be completed differently to the open first round. Example of a Round 2 cover letter is included in Figure 5.1. This letter is again taken from the same study used to illustrate the Round 1 information pack.

Dear **Expert Panel Member**

Re: Study Name

Thank you for returning the first round Delphi questionnaire. You will now find enclosed the second round Delphi questionnaire which includes all the responses from your profession in relation to research priorities.

You will find enclosed with this letter an instruction sheet and the second-round Delphi questionnaire. This questionnaire is completed differently to the first round and the instruction sheet will guide you through this process. Please read the instructions carefully and complete the Delphi questionnaire as fully as you can. Return of completed Delphi Round 2 implies consent to participate.

If you could return the questionnaire in the enclosed stamped addressed envelope or by e-mail to **insert researcher's e-mail address** by **insert return date**, we would be most grateful. If you wish to discuss any aspect of this further, please contact **researcher's contact details**.

Thank you for your continued participation in this study.

Yours sincerely,
Principal Investigator

Figure 5.1   Example of cover letter for Round 2 classical Delphi

Instructions for Round 2

An example of the type of instructions which should be sent to the expert panel is included in Figure 5.2. If using a modified Delphi technique, then the cover letter and instructions illustrated in Figures 5.1 and 5.2 could be modified for use in the first written Delphi round after the modification (e.g. focus groups or interviews).

Instructions on how to complete Delphi Round 2

The second round of this Delphi lists all the responses from panel members in Round 1. These responses have been content analysed and similar responses grouped together to ensure that the questionnaire is not repetitive and easily completed. The meaning of the responses has not been changed.

You will see a scale beside each research topic. This scale is numbered 1 to 5. Please place an X in the box which you feel best describes how important the research topic is. These numbers correspond to a response as below:

1 – Very Important
2 – Important
3 – Neither important or not important
4 – Not important
5 – Unimportant

Once you have completed the questionnaire, please return it to the researcher in the enclosed stamped addressed envelope or by e-mail to **insert e-mail address** by **insert return date**.

Figure 5.2   Example of instructions for Round 2

Delphi Round Two

Please place an X in the box which you feel best describes how important the research topic is. These numbers correspond to a response as below:

1 – Very Important

2 – Important

3 – Neither important or not important

4 – Not important

5 – Unimportant

Research Topic	1 2 3 4 5
	☐ ☐ ☐ ☐ ☐
	☐ ☐ ☐ ☐ ☐
	☐ ☐ ☐ ☐ ☐
	☐ ☐ ☐ ☐ ☐
	☐ ☐ ☐ ☐ ☐
	☐ ☐ ☐ ☐ ☐
	☐ ☐ ☐ ☐ ☐
	☐ ☐ ☐ ☐ ☐
	☐ ☐ ☐ ☐ ☐

Figure 5.3   Example of layout of Round Two classical Delphi questionnaire

Designing Round 2 questionnaires

The layout of a Round 2 questionnaire used within the classical Delphi technique is illustrated at Figure 5.3. Obviously, there are many variations in the way that a Round 2 Delphi questionnaire can be designed. However, all these types of layouts will have certain common features:

1. Statements or items for ranking or rating.
2. A scale of some description for ranking or rating purposes, such as a numerical scale or a 'strongly agree' to 'strongly disagree' textual scale or 'most important' to 'least important' textual scale.

Sometimes it can be useful to group the analysed statements from Round 1 into categories to allow the expert panel member to see statements within the same general area together to consider their importance or agreement with in that context. It can also serve to split up the questionnaire and make it easier and more visually appealing to the expert panel member to complete.

Likert scales

A Likert scale is a psychometric scale commonly used in all types of questionnaires and is the most widely used scale in survey research in all disciplines. It is generally used in questionnaires to facilitate respondents to indicate their level of agreement with a statement. This makes the Likert scale a perfect scale to use within a Delphi questionnaire as the technique is most concerned with agreement and consensus. A typical 5-point Likert scale is illustrated in Figure 5.3 in the Round 2 example of a Delphi questionnaire.

Round 2 analysis

Data from returned Round 2 questionnaires should be input into SPSS (Statistical Package for the Social Scientists), for analysis or a similar statistical analysis package. Summary statistics (frequencies; descriptives) should be run on the data to determine the number of statements that have reached consensus at this stage (for example greater than 70% agreement or whatever consensus level has been previously agreed). Statements that have reached consensus can be eliminated from Round 3 at this stage. This does not mean that these are the highest research priorities, merely that they have reached consensus first. However, some researchers choose to include all statements again at Round 3 even those that have already reached consensus. There are advantages and disadvantages of this approach. The advantages are that all statements receive an equal chance to gain consensus at the highest possible level. The disadvantages are that the questionnaires will not become shorter as rounds go on and the risk of losing expert panel members becomes greater. The decision again must be balanced between keeping the response rate high enough to have a viable study and gaining consensus at the highest level. If there are only a small number of statements generated at Round 1, then the best approach would be to include all statements the whole way through the process. If large and unmanageable amounts of statements are generated at Round 2, it may be prudent to take statements off as consensus is reached. It is useful then to include a summary sheet of statements already at consensus with subsequent rounds to serve as feedback to the expert panel. It could also serve to stimulate their interest in the study and their continued participation. As every Delphi study is different and has different issues, these decisions must be made as the study progresses.

The ranking of research priorities overall does not happen until the end of the Delphi process. Further detail on analysis of the statistical rounds of the Delphi will be provided in Chapter 6.

Sample motivation

It is important in a Delphi study to keep the expert panel motivated and interested enough to complete and return all the Delphi rounds that are sent to them. This can be achieved by keeping the panel up to date with the progress of the Delphi, for example appraising them of items that have gained consensus already or sending them a progress report on the study with their packs. Keeping the sample motivated is key to gaining a high response rate in each round (Sandrey & Bulger, 2008). This is generally more difficult with a large sample and easier with a small sample.

Follow-ups/reminders

Follow-ups are very important when using the Delphi technique as with any survey method. Normally, reminders are written in the form of a letter or postcard but with the Delphi technique reminders have also been given by telephone or e-mail due to the nature of the researcher knowing who each panel member is. A fuller explanation of the use of reminders or follow-ups is included in Chapter 5. Reminders are a good way of enhancing the response rates in each round (Dillman, 1978; Edwards *et al.*, 2002).

Round 3

Round 3 should be designed using the rated or ranked items from Round 2. As before expert panel members should be sent a cover letter (see Figure 5.4), a set of instructions for Round 3 (see Figure 5.5), the Round 3 questionnaire (see Figure 5.6) and an SAE. Round 3 of the Delphi, as with Round 2, should be designed to provide feedback to the expert on the statements to date and to provide an opportunity for panel members to change their response from Round 2.

As within the previous rounds, expert panel members will be asked to return the completed questionnaire within the given time period using the enclosed SAE or by email if using an e-Delphi approach. The master codes continue to link each expert panel members' responses to each round. Again, follow-up reminders will be sent to expert panel members as necessary.

Individual and group feedback

Round 3 in the classical Delphi technique is the stage whereby expert panel members can begin to converge on consensus. Statements that have

Dear **Expert Panel Member**

Re: Study Name

Thank you for returning the second round Delphi questionnaire. You will now find enclosed the third round Delphi questionnaire which includes details on the research topics that you have been involved in identifying and rating in relation to importance. You will also find enclosed a list of the research priorities that have already reached consensus on their importance. This does not mean that they are the most important priorities, only that they have reached consensus at an early stage.

You will find enclosed with this letter an instruction sheet and the third round Delphi questionnaire. As before, this questionnaire is completed differently to the first and second round questionnaires and the instruction sheet enclosed will guide you through this process.

Please read the instructions carefully and complete the Delphi questionnaire as fully as you can. Return of completed Delphi Round 3 implies consent to participate.

If you could return the questionnaire in the enclosed stamped addressed envelope or by email to **insert e-mail address** by **insert return date,** we would be most grateful. If you wish to discuss any aspect of this further, please contact **insert researcher's details**.

Thank you for your continued participation in this study.

Yours sincerely,
Principal Investigator

Figure 5.4   **Example of cover letter for classical Delphi Round 3**

Instructions on how to complete Delphi Round 3

The third round of this Delphi includes those research topics that have not yet reached agreement from the panel on their importance. You will see three columns beside each statement.

Column one shows the group response to the research topic. This will appear as a number which corresponds to the same scale as in Round 2 and which is outlined below. Column two shows your own individual response to the research topic. Again this will appear as a number which corresponds to the scale below:

1 – Very Important
2 – Important
3 – Neither important or not important
4 – Not important
5 – Unimportant

Column three is blank and is provided as an opportunity for you to reconsider your response since Round 2. We would appreciate it if you would reconsider your original response in the context of the group response to each benchmark and if you wish to change your response, please do so by placing an X in the appropriate box beside each benchmark. Please note that you do not have to change your original response if you do not wish to.

Once you have completed the questionnaire, please return it to the researcher in the enclosed stamped addressed envelope or by email to **insert e-mail address** by **insert return date**.

Figure 5.5   **Example of instructions for classical Delphi Round 3**

Delphi Round Three

Please reconsider your response in the context of the feedback provided. If you wish to change your response, please place an X in the box which you feel best describes how important the research topic is. These numbers correspond to a response as below:

1 – Very Important

2 – Important

3 – Neither important or not important

4 – Not important

5 – Unimportant

Statement	Your Response from Round 2	Overall Group Response	New Response
			1 2 3 4 5
			☐ ☐☐☐ ☐
			☐ ☐☐☐ ☐
			☐ ☐☐☐ ☐
			☐ ☐☐☐ ☐
			☐ ☐☐☐ ☐
			☐ ☐☐☐ ☐
			☐ ☐☐☐ ☐
			☐ ☐☐☐ ☐

Figure 5.6   Example of Round three questionnaire for classical Delphi approach

not yet reached consensus (and possibly all statements as discussed above) are presented again and three columns of information are provided beside each statement:

1. The individual response from the last round, for example very important

2. The group response (median), for example not important
3. A space for the individual to change their response, for example not important

An example of the layout of a Round 3 Delphi questionnaire is included at Figure 5.6. This is the third round questionnaire from the same study used to illustrate Rounds 1 and 2.

Round 3 analysis

If Round 3 is the last round of the Delphi process for the study, overall analysis is undertaken at this stage. If there is to be a Round 4 (for example if consensus has not been reached on sufficient items), the same process as outlined for Round 3 would be undertaken. For many studies, three Delphi rounds are sufficient. Overall final analysis entails the entering of Round 3 data into SPSS. As before, frequencies and descriptives should be run on the data to determine the number of statements that have reached consensus at this stage (e.g. greater than 70% agreement or whatever has been determined at the outset of the study).

The statements that have gained consensus should form the final list of research priorities. The mean of each of these statements should be calculated and used to rank the statements in order from most important to least important. Generally in a research priorities Delphi, this will result in a list of at least the top ten research priorities for the specific area in which the Delphi is being undertaken. Further detail on analysis of all statistical rounds of the Delphi can be found in Chapter 6.

Number of rounds

One of the basic principles underpinning the Delphi technique is to have as many rounds as are required to achieve consensus or until the law of diminishing returns occurs (McKenna, 1994a). Provision for feedback and opportunity to revise earlier responses obviously requires that the Delphi has at least two rounds. However, the number of rounds can be a matter of dispute. Although there are no strict guidelines on the correct number of rounds, as discussed in Chapters 1 and 2, the number can depend upon the time available and whether the researcher ignited the Delphi sequence with one broad question or with a list of questions or events. In addressing the law of diminishing returns (McKenna, 1994a), the number of rounds may be decreased to minimise reductions in the amount of new information and reductions in response rates resulting from respondent fatigue (Starkweather *et al.*, 1975).

When to stop

There are several factors to consider when decided when to stop the rounds of a Delphi questionnaire. For example, if in Round 2, all items gain consensus, then that would be the time to stop. However, this would be a rare occurrence. Usually, the decision on when to stop is not as straight-forward as this and usually has to be taken after Round 3. The normal dilemma is that many statements have gained consensus but some still have not after three rounds, the response rate is dwindling and the expert panel is losing interest and motivation. A decision has to be made between the importance of gaining consensus on all items and the importance of maintaining a high response rate. Usually, Delphi researchers will accept that some items are not going to gain consensus after three rounds and will stop the technique at this point. Sometimes the items that do not gain consensus are as important in terms of findings as those items that do gain consensus.

When not to stop

When an expert panel is highly motivated and interested in the issue being investigated, this is a perfect opportunity to continue administering Delphi rounds until consensus is gained on as many items as possible. This usually only happens in Delphi studies that have small expert panels who are experts in an extremely focussed field.

Reaching consensus

It should be noted that the existence of consensus from a Delphi process does not mean that the correct answer has been found (Keeney *et al.*, 2001, 2006). This method is not a replacement for rigorous scientific reviews of published reports or for original research. There is a danger that the 'Delphi' can lead the observer to place greater reliance on their results than might otherwise be warranted. In addition, the Delphi has been criticised as a method which forces consensus and is weakened by not allowing participants to discuss issues, so no opportunity arises for respondents to elaborate on their views (Goodman, 1987; Walker & Selfe, 1996). However, as long as this is kept in mind and addressed, consensus can be gained and the Delphi can be used as a useful, integral consensus technique (Keeney *et al.*, 2006).

It is apparent that there is no universal agreement on what the level of consensus for a Delphi study should be, or how this level of consensus should be decided. In conclusion, this must be a decision for each Delphi researcher to make in consultation with the literature and the conviction that consensus is reached when the researcher's pre-determined level of consensus (e.g. 70%) is gained on a specific item or topic.

Key learning points

- The Delphi technique employs a number of rounds in which questionnaires are sent out until consensus is reached.
- Round 1 of the classical Delphi begins with an open-ended round allowing panels freedom in their responses.
- Round 1 is generally an idea-generation round.
- It is important to send information packs with each round of the Delphi giving clear instructions to the expert panel members.
- In a modified Delphi, the open-ended first round does not normally take place; modifications can include using the literature to formulate statements, using focus groups or one-to-one interviews.
- Careful consideration should be given to the number of items that expert panel members can identify in an open-ended first round as this has implications for the length of Round 2 and three questionnaires.
- Rounds 2 and other subsequent rounds take the form of structured questionnaires, usually with Likert scales to allow expert panel members to rate or rank statements.
- Round 3 and subsequent rounds give feedback to the expert panel in the form of both individual feedback and group feedback.
- An item has reached consensus when the pre-determined level (e.g. 70%) has been reached; that is 70% of the sample is in agreement with how important that statement is.
- The law of diminishing returns should be considered when deciding when to stop the rounds of the Delphi.

Recommended further reading

Beretta, R. (1996) A critical review of the Delphi Technique. *Nurse Researcher* 3(4), 79–89.

Burnard, P. (1991) A method of analysing interview transcripts in qualitative research. *Nurse Education Today* 11(6), 461–466.

McKenna, H.P. (1994) The Delphi technique: a worthwhile approach for nursing? *Journal of Advanced Nursing* 19, 1221–1225.

6 Analysing Data from a Delphi and Reporting Results

Introduction

This chapter will describe the process of analysing data from the classical Delphi technique based on a three round approach. Other types of Delphi, for example the modified Delphi can also follow this process for the rounds included in the approach as necessary.

In the Delphi process, data analysis involves both qualitative and quantitative data if the classical approach is used. Qualitative data is analysed after the first round of the process, which uses open-ended questions to collect expert opinion. This is discussed in Chapters 4 and 5. Subsequent rounds are used to identify and achieve the desired level of consensus as well as any changes of judgements among panellists (Hsu & Sandford, 2007).

The main statistics used in Delphi studies are measures of central tendency (mean, median and mode) and level of dispersion (standard deviation and inter-quartile range) in order to present information concerning the collective judgements of respondents (Hasson *et al.*, 2000). Generally, the uses of median and mode are favoured. However, in some cases, the mean is used (Murray & Jarman, 1987). Use of the mean, however, has been questioned by some Delphi researchers. Witkin (1984) queried the appropriateness of using the mean to measure the subjects' responses if scales used in Delphi studies are not delineated at equal intervals. In the literature, the use of the median, based on Likert-type scale, is strongly favoured to provide feedback to the expert panel (Hill & Fowles, 1975; Eckman, 1983; Jacobs, 1996). Jacobs (1996) stated 'considering the anticipated consensus of opinion and the skewed expectation of responses as they were compiled, the median would inherently appear best suited to reflect the resultant convergence of opinion' (p. 57).

Analysis of Round 1

Content analysis – the practical aspects

Round 1 of the classical Delphi is a qualitative round as discussed in the previous chapters. The open-ended nature of this round means that the method of analysis used is a qualitative approach, namely content analysis. Chapter 5 also discusses the types of content analysis that could be used.

The method of content analysis used can vary from study to study and is generally at the discretion of the researcher. While the data is themed in the same manner as unstructured qualitative data, the process differs slightly in that the statements provided by the expert panel in Round 1 should remain as true to the wording as possible.

All statements from the returned Round 1 questionnaire should be typed into a word processing document to allow for cutting and pasting and moving statements in under themes. The process really begins with the identification of statements that are either the same or so similar that they mean the same thing. These statements should be grouped together and themes developed around similar statements and statements that are in the same area of interest.

Once statements that are the same or very similar are all grouped together, the researcher should make a decision on whether these statements should be collapsed into one statement, and if so, what wording to use. In this case, wording should be kept as true to one of the statements provided by the expert panel. The other statements should then be discarded.

Unique statements, that is statements provided by the expert panel with nothing similar emerging, should be kept as worded and included directly in Round 2.

Once all similar statements have been collapsed and put with the unique statements, it is useful to organise the final list of statements into themes. This allows the researcher to have insight into the broad areas in which statements are being identified by the expert panel. It is also a useful way to organise the Round 2 questionnaire as discussed in Chapter 5.

It is worth considering the length of time that this process will take when estimating how quickly the Delphi process will proceed. The more expert panel members there are, the more statements are likely to be generated. This can create a large and unwieldy amount of data which could produce many similar but not exactly the same types of statements. The researcher should consider the nature and profile of the expert panel in deciding on how specific to keep the statements or on how rigorously to collapse them. It is sometimes useful to share the anonymised raw data, and the final collapsed list with another member of the team to ensure the collapsing process has not changed the meaning of any of the statements. After this process, the Round 2 questionnaire should be designed, using this final list of statements.

Demographics for sample profiling

If demographic data are collected as part of the Round 1 process, then this data should be analysed at this stage to give an overall profile of the expert panel. An example of the type of demographic data that could be collected from the expert panel is included in Chapter 5. It is not essential to collect this type of data within the Delphi process, especially if the members of the expert panel are well known to the researcher. However, it does provide an opportunity to describe the expert panel and their experience.

A Statistical Package for the Social Scientists (SPSS) database should be set up using the demographic labels as variables. For example, age, gender, years experience in profession, number of publications in the area. Data should be inputted into SPSS for each expert panel member linked to their master code. Frequencies and descriptives can be undertaken on the data to provide percentages of males and females in the sample or the mean age of the sample or whatever analysis is appropriate for the particular expert panel included in the study. Delphi researchers should familiarise themselves with SPSS (Field, 2005; Pallant, 2007), or a similar statistical software package to analyse the results from the closed rounds of a Delphi regardless of which type of Delphi is used. SPSS will be used as the software package to illustrate analysis within this chapter.

Analysis of middle rounds (Round 2)

Consensus level

The consensus level will have been decided by the researcher or research team at the outset of the study and will be important when considering the returned Round 2 questionnaire responses.

Statistical analysis

When Round 2 questionnaires have all been returned or the return date and reminder processes have been completed, an SPSS database should be set up for the analysis of the Round 2 data. Each statement should be set up as a separate variable in SPSS. Responses from each expert panel should be inputted to the SPSS database alongside their master code. More information on master codes is included in Chapter 5.

Once all the data from the Round 2 questionnaires has been inputted, frequencies should be run on the entire dataset. This will provide output on the percentage of each overall response to each statement. For example, see Table 6.1. This shows a frequency table from a Delphi study after Round 2. Expert panel members were asked to rate the statement 'Research into models of care, e.g. primary care versus secondary care for musculoskeletal outpatients department' as an 'important' or

Table 6.1   Example of frequency output from SPSS

Research into models of care, e.g. primary care versus secondary care for musculoskeletal outpatient departments					
		Frequency	Per cent	Valid per cent	Cumulative per cent
Valid	Very unimportant	1	1.8	1.8	1.8
	Quite unimportant	3	5.5	5.5	7.3
	Neither	17	30.9	30.9	38.2
	Quite important	26	47.3	47.3	85.5
	Very important	8	14.5	14.5	100.0
	Total	55	100.0	100.0	

'unimportant' research priority. Table 6.1 shows that the statement has not reached the consensus level of 70% as pre-determined at the start of the study but that 47.3% of the expert panel have rated it as 'quite important' and 14.5% have rated it as 'very important'. This statement will be sent out again as part of the Round 3 questionnaire and has a good change of gaining a consensus level of 70% if some members of the expert panel change their response.

Statistical feedback to panel

To encourage convergence on consensus, expert panel members are given individual and group feedback within the Round 3 questionnaire. An example of the design of a Round 3 questionnaire is included in Chapter 6. This feedback is normally provided using the median. Descriptive statistics should be undertaken on the Round 2 SPSS database to determine the median and in some cases researchers also calculate the standard deviation to examine the range of responses. The standard deviation can also be included in feedback to the expert panel in Round 3 if the researcher wishes to do so. The standard deviation would be used in feedback to show the spread of responses from the expert panel. Table 6.2 shows the

Table 6.2   Example of descriptive output from SPSS

Statistics		
Research into models of care, e.g. primary care versus secondary care for musculoskeletal outpatient departments		
N	Valid	55
	Missing	0
Median		4.00
Standard deviation		0.862

SPSS output for the same statement including the mean and the standard deviation. The likert scale used in these examples is as follows:

1. Very Unimportant
2. Quite Unimportant
3. Neither Important or Unimportant
4. Quite Important
5. Very Important

The output shows that the median for this statement is 4 which is 'quite important' and the standard deviation is 0.862. Therefore, the feedback given to the expert panel at Round 3 will be that the majority of the sample at this stage of the process have rated this statements as 4 on a scale of 1–5 which equates to 'quite important'. Each expert panel member will also be reminded of their own response which could be, for example 3 – 'neither important or unimportant' and in the light of the group response could be persuaded to consider the statement again and change their response to 4 – 'quite important', thus moving the statement further towards the 70% target for consensus.

Exclusion of items with consensus

Some statements may gain consensus at Round 2, that is 70% of the expert panel agree on the importance or ranking position of the statement. Some Delphi researchers have advocated removing these statements from the Round 3 questionnaire and 'banking' them as having already gained consensus. These statements are then flagged up to the expert panel as having already reached consensus and are set apart from the statements included in the Round 3 questionnaire. The statements that have not yet reached consensus are included in the Round 3 questionnaire and the expert panel are asked to re-consider their response in the light of the group response.

There are some advantages and disadvantages in adopting this approach. On the positive side, excluding the statements that have already reached consensus shortens the Round 3 questionnaire and may encourage the expert panel to complete it if it is shorter. The feedback of statements that have already reached consensus may help motivate the expert panel as they can see that the process has actually worked. However, on a more negative note, the statements that did not gain consensus and that are sent out again at Round 3 have an opportunity to gain a higher level of consensus than those statements removed after Round 2 and possibly a higher rating of importance. By keeping all statements in for all three rounds of the classical Delphi, every statement is getting an equal chance to gain the highest importance rating and level of consensus as each other. As with many aspects of the Delphi technique this is a decision that has to be made by the researcher when considering all factors pertaining to their specific Delphi study.

Analysis of end round (Round 3)

Determining the end of the process

In the classical Delphi, Round 3 would usually be the end of the process. However, some studies do require a Round 4. If there were very few statements that had gained consensus by Round 3, the researcher may be left with no option but to undertake as further round. If that is the case, the same instructions and analysis described for Round 3 would apply to Round 4. Generally, by the end of Round 3, a lot of statements will have reached consensus and most researchers will stop at that point. Statements that have not reached consensus at this stage are sometimes just as interesting as statements that have reached consensus in terms of findings.

Statistical analysis

When all Round 3 questionnaires have been returned or the return date and reminder processes have been completed, an SPSS database should be set up for the analysis of the Round 3 data. As before, each statement should be used as a variable in SPSS. Responses from each expert panel should be inputted to the SPSS database alongside their master code. This could be done in the same database containing Round 2 results as long as the statements are carefully labelled Round 2 and Round 3. Sometimes it is more helpful to have separate databases linked by master codes for each expert panel member.

Once all the data from the Round 3 questionnaires has been inputted, frequencies should be run on the entire dataset. This will provide output on the percentage of each overall response to each statement. For example see Table 6.3. This shows a frequency table from a Delphi study after Round 3.

Expert panel members were asked to rate the statement 'A study to assess the clinical effectiveness of manual therapy and establish optimal treatment parameters' as an important or unimportant research priority.

Table 6.3   Example of frequency output for Round 3

A study to assess the clinical effectiveness of manual therapy and establish optimal treatment parameters				
		Frequency	Per cent	Valid per cent	Cumulative per cent
Valid	Very unimportant	1	1.8	1.8	1.8
	Quite unimportant	7	9.4	9.4	11.2
	Neither	8	0.0	0.0	11.2
	Quite important	28	14.5	14.5	25.7
	Very important	11	74.3	74.3	100.0
	Total	55	100.0	100.0	

Table 6.3 shows that the statement reached consensus after three rounds at 74.3%. This means that 74.3% of the expert panel has agreed that the statement is 'very important'. This is known as the level of agreement on the statement. However, this does not determine the level of importance of the statement within the context of all the statements rated in the three rounds of the Delphi process. The level of importance of the statement is calculated using the mean.

Items that have gained consensus

Statements that have reached consensus should have their mean calculated using the SPSS Round 3 database, and the mean should then be used to rank the statements in order of importance. Table 6.4 shows an example of an SPSS descriptives table outlining the mean of each statement. Table 6.5 shows these statements ranked by the mean (importance rating) alongside their level of consensus (level of agreement).

Items that have not gained consensus

At the end of the Delphi process, there is no doubt that not all of the statements will have gained consensus. Some statements may be very near consensus and others may be far from consensus. While many studies do not report on the statements that did not gain consensus, these statements should be examined as they can reveal interesting findings. Researchers should consider why these statements did not gain consensus; are there

Table 6.4   Example of an SPSS descriptives table at Round 3 of a Delphi study

Descriptive statistics		
	N	**Mean**
Conduct an evaluation of needs and access of conditions, e.g. Parkinson's disease	7	4.02
Research into patient/carer views of service providers	7	3.93
Research into patient attendance, including self referral and DNA rates for particular groups and conditions	7	3.67
Research the differences between treatment in public and private health care systems	7	3.38
Research the role of the physiotherapist in preventive medicine/keeping people out of hospital	7	4.25
Role of physiotherapist as first contact practitioner for musculoskeletal disorders	7	4.13
Identify areas of service inequality for post-neurological trauma across a geographical/population basis	7	3.85
Valid *N* (listwise)	7	

Table 6.5   Statements that have gained consensus ranked by mean (level of importance)

Statement	Mean	Consensus level
Research the role of the physiotherapist in PCCC in preventive medicine/keeping people out of hospital	4.25	85%
Research the role of the physiotherapist as first contact practitioner for musculoskeletal disorders	4.13	87%
Conduct an evaluation of needs and access to services for a range of conditions, e.g. Parkinson's disease	4.02	76%
Research into patient/carer views of service providers	3.93	75%
Identify areas of service inequity for post-neurological trauma across a geographical population basis	3.85	72%
Research into patient attendance, including self-referral and DNA rates for particular groups and conditions	3.67	72%
Research the differences between treatment in public and private health care systems	3.38	70%

any particular reasons to explain this? It may also be interesting for an expert panel to receive feedback on the statements that did not achieve consensus.

Stability of responses

The stability of responses within a Delphi study is not often reported in resulting reports or publications. However, they can be important if the stability of each individual's responses is a factor which you want to report in your study (Greatorex & Dexter, 2000). Greatorex and Dexter (2000) described in great detail the process of what happens between the rounds of a Delphi and comment on the stability of responses across the rounds. For Delphi studies where the scale on which the expert panel are asked to indicate their opinion is considered to be interval, the mean or median are used to represent group opinion and the standard deviation used to indicate the level of agreement. Some methodological publications do report upon what happens between the rounds of the Delphi in detail and are worth consulting if interested in this specific area of Delphi methodology (Scheibe *et al.*, 1975; Erffmeyer *et al.*, 1986; Taylor *et al.*, 1990; Martino, 1993). Scheibe *et al.* (1975) stated that, in their opinion, the use of percentages alone is inadequate in relation to Delphi analysis. They suggested that a more reliable alternative is to measure the stability of subjects' responses in successive iterations. Dajani *et al.* (1979) proposed that the chi-square test was used to test the stability of group responses between rounds. They believed that group stability had occurred if there was no significant difference between the frequencies for the responses for two consecutive Delphi rounds. Chaffin and Talley's (1980) paper on individual stability sets out exactly how to use chi-square for this purpose.

The main method advocated in the recent literature for determining stability across responses is the use of Kappa statistics (Holey *et al.*, 2007). Stability refers to the 'within-subject' level of agreement in the expert panel member's responses to two rounds. It does not refer to the level of agreement between expert panel members. SPSS will calculate non-weighted Kappa statistics. For a full explanation of the Kappa statistics and how to use it to determine stability of each panel members responses across the rounds, see Chaffin and Talley (1980).

Examples of statistical analysis used in recent Delphi studies

Many published Delphi studies are not explicit in resultant publications about the statistical tests used to analyse responses or to provide feedback. It is also evident within those publications that do specify statistical tests that there is wide variation in which statistics are used. Table 6.6 outlines some recent Delphi studies and the types of statistical analysis they used for Rounds 2 and 3 of the Delphi process.

Reporting of results from a Delphi study

Most published Delphi studies focus primarily upon the findings. However, according to Evans (1997), the terms agreement and consensus are essentially two different ideologies. Is there a difference between the extent to which each participant agrees with the *issue* under consideration and the extent to which participants agree with *each other*? When reporting findings, few studies do so in the context of these different principles. Most researchers prefer instead to rely upon participants agreeing with *each other*. Yet it is important to note that the extent to which participants agree with each other does not mean that consensus exists nor does it mean that the 'correct' answer has been found. This is especially the case when the issues have ethical implications. For example, 75% of a nursing panel may agree that very old and ill patients should not be put through the rigours of active resuscitation. This reflects consensus in the Delphi sense, but it may not be the correct way to care for such patients. It is important to remember that the results from a Delphi study are 'specific to the panel of experts' (Sandrey & Bulger, 2008, p. 137).

A panel member may be reluctant to share a view contrary to the majority of panel members. However, this is how the Delphi works. It is only through seeing the (anonymised) responses from other panel members that individual participants are encouraged to reconsider their views. Delphi purists would argue that panel members change their minds and move towards consensus because they see that someone else has identified a more relevant issue that they had not thought of. Delphi cynics would assert that panel members are cajoled to change their minds because of a possible mistaken belief that the views expressed by the majority of the

Table 6.6 Examples of statistical analysis used in published studies

Authors and year	Subject of paper	Type of Delphi	Statistical analysis used for Rounds 2 and 3	Statistics used to provide feedback
Vogel *et al.* (2009)	Prevention of adolescents' music-induced hearing loss due to discotheque attendance: a Delphi study	Online Delphi 3 rounds	Percentages, median and inter-quartile range	Median and inter-quartile range
Becker *et al.* (2009)	Do we agree? Using a Delphi technique to develop consensus on skills of hand expression	Classical Delphi 3 rounds	Percentages, median and inter-quartile range	Median and inter-quartile range
Ferguson *et al.* (2008)	A Delphi study investigating consensus among expert physiotherapists in relation to management of low back pain	Classical Delphi 3 rounds	Percentages and mean	Not specified
Drennan *et al.* (2007)	Nursing Research Priorities	Decision Delphi 3 rounds and consensus conference	Percentages, mean and standard deviation	Mean and standard deviation
Efstathiou *et al.* (2007)	Healthcare providers' priorities for cancer care	Classical Delphi 3 rounds	Percentages, mean, standard deviation, correlation coefficients, Kruskal Wallis and Kendall's W	Mean and standard deviation
Susic *et al.* (2006)	Community actions against alcohol drinking in Slovenia	Classical Delphi 3 rounds	Percentages and mean	Mean
Avery *et al.* (2005)	Identifying and establishing consensus on the most important safety features of GP computer systems	e-Delphi 2 rounds	Percentages and median	Median

(*Continued*)

Table 6.6 (*Continued*)

Authors and year	Subject of paper	Type of Delphi	Statistical analysis used for Rounds 2 and 3	Statistics used to provide feedback
Madigan & Vanderboom (2005)	Home health care nursing research priorities	Classical Delphi 3 rounds	Percentages, mean and standard deviation	Mean and standard deviation
McBride *et al.* (2003)	Delphi survey of experts opinions on strategies used by community pharmacists to reduce over the counter drug misuse	Modified Delphi Interviews and 3 rounds	Percentages, median and inter-quartile range	Median and inter-quartile range
Sowell (2000)	Identifying HIV/AIDS research priorities for the next millennium	Classical Delphi 3 rounds	Percentages, mean, standard deviation and chi-square	Mean and standard deviation
Dwyer (1999)	A Delphi study of research priorities and identified areas for collaborative research in health library and information services UK	Classical Delphi 3 rounds	Percentages, median and inter-quartile range	Median and inter-quartile range

panel must be right. The obvious conclusion of this assertion is that strong-willed panel members hold rigidly to their views across rounds and weak-willed panel members alter theirs. If true, this challenges seriously the validity and reliability of Delphi findings.

Therefore, it is clear that there is a danger of placing too much reliance upon the final results without acknowledging the influence of bias and other factors on validity and reliability (see Chapter 7). To enhance authenticity, a number of strategies can be used. For instance, pilot testing could be undertaken (Mitchell, 1991; Gordon, 1994; Miller, 2001; Novakowski & Wellar, 2008), the integration of an additional methodological technique, such as focus groups or interviews (McKenna, 1994b), or the comparison with secondary validated data.

Key learning points

- In the Delphi process, data analysis involves both qualitative and quantitative data if the classical approach is used.
- The main statistics used in Delphi studies are measures of central tendency (mean, median and mode) and level of dispersion (standard deviation and inter-quartile range) in order to present information concerning the collective judgements of respondents (Hasson *et al.*, 2000).
- Round 1 of the classical Delphi is a qualitative round as discussed in the previous chapters. The open-ended nature of this round means that the method of analysis used is a qualitative approach, namely content analysis (see Chapter 5 for more detail on content analysis).
- The SPSS is frequently used to analyse the statistical data from a Delphi study.
- To encourage convergence on consensus, expert panel members are given individual and group feedback with each new questionnaire that they are sent.
- The stability of responses within a Delphi study is not often reported in resulting reports or publications. However, they can be important if the stability of each individual's responses is a factor which you want to report in your study. For further information on stability, see Chafin and Talley (1980) included in reference list.

Recommended further reading

Chafin, V.W. & Talley, W.K. (1980) Individual stability in Delphi studies. *Technological Forecasting and Social Change* 16, 67–73.

Hasson, F., Keeney, S. & McKenna, H.P. (2000) Research guidelines for the Delphi technique. *Journal of Advanced Nursing* 32(4), 1008–1015.

Hsu, C.C. & Sandford, B.A. (2007) The Delphi technique: making sense of consensus. *Practical Assessment, Research and Evaluation* 12(10), 1–8.

7 Reliability and Validity

Introduction

Similar to all types of inquiry, establishing methodological rigour is vital to the integrity of research; the Delphi technique is no different. However, establishing this, for the Delphi technique, is not straightforward for a number of reasons. Firstly, the ongoing debate concerning the epistemological paradigm within which the Delphi technique fits raises many dilemmas, particularly as conventional wisdom believes the transference of terms across paradigms is inappropriate. The terms 'validity and reliability' within the positivist quantitative approach, have been argued in the literature as not being pertinent to qualitative inquiry (Altheide & Johnson, 1994). Yet, the juxtaposition of the technique between the positivist and naturalistic paradigms raises a problem on which standards to adopt. Secondly, the continual modifications of the technique make the process of testing problematic. Consequently, the number of studies exploring rigour is scant, many outdated and made-up of experimental Delphi studies that attempt to isolate and test a particular component of the method (Crisp et al., 1997). The majority of early research has focused on demonstrating rigour from a mainly quantitative position only a handful of recent examples have started to give credence to the qualitative paradigm. This chapter aims to present a brief discussion of the principal forms of establishing rigour, using the Delphi technique; early examples are cited, however, for an in-depth analysis of early studies, the reader is advised to refer to Woudenber (1991) and Rowe et al. (1991) reviews.

Reliability

Reliability refers to an examination of stability and equivalence of the research conditions and procedures. Unlike other approaches, it is assumed the Delphi approach enhances reliability two main ways. Firstly, by the decision-making process, as participants do not need to meet

The Delphi Technique in Nursing and Health Research, First Edition, © S. Keeney,
F. Hasson and H. McKenna   Published 2011 by Blackwell Publishing Ltd.

face-to-face therefore avoiding group bias and group think scenarios and secondly, as the panel size increases the reliability of the respondent group also grows. Although a number of writers question this claim (Sackman, 1975; Rowe *et al.*, 1991; Woudenberg, 1991; Williams & Webb, 1994b; Yousuf, 2007a), proposing that measures obtained from judgements are questionable; one of the most common indicators of reliability is the test-retest method, which measures the consistency of results over different timeframes. In an early study, Uhl (1975) gave 26 faculty members a questionnaire consisting of 110 items asking their perception of the degree of importance given by their institution to various goals and as well as their opinion on the degree of importance. Despite wide divergence, consensus was obtained in three rounds. To test reliability, a year later the same panel were given the same questionnaire, results were found to be significantly like the initial Delphi round than the final one. Consensus originally gained did not seem to be long lasting, questioning the reliability of the technique.

Reliability has also been measured by comparing two groups of participants' results in the same Delphi. For example in 1964, Ament (1970) conducted a Delphi study on the long-range forecasting of scientific and technological developments; he then repeated it in 1969 using a different set of experts. Whilst he found that items predicted by panellists to occur in 10 years before 1980, shifted further into the future, he did find forecasting behaviours to be similar despite a 5-year gap. In 1968, Helmer compared the results across three different Delphi studies conducted in 1964, 1966 and 1967. The first study was conducted using a traditional Delphi design, the second a pre-test which involved 23 Rand Corporation employees, and the final was undertaken at a conference with 100 conference delegates, of which 23 were selected to participate with no anonymity guaranteed. The 1963 study presented four questions related but not identical to the other two studies, concern over question-wording, caused conference delegates to raise concern about bias and unreliability of their results. Only one event was forecasted to occur in the same year by two groups and six other forecasts differed in 2- to 9-year timeframe. Correlation coefficient presented by Helmer was 0.87. In a review, Wondenberg (1991) strongly criticised the lack of similarity between the studies viewing the calculation of coefficient as a pointless exercise.

A number of studies have compared panel's results, from studies that have started with the same information and included experts with similar characteristics. For example Welty (1971, 1972), although he aimed to discredit the Delphi's claim for the need for experts by comparing judgements between experts and laypeople, also found that the method was reliable. In the both studies, participants were asked to estimate on a five-point scale the importance of various American cultural issues. Results from the first study showed no significant differences ($p = 0.18$) and in the second study, results were only significantly different on two issues, leading him to claim that high levels of expertise are not required and that, in fact, the method is reliable. Yet such claims have been refuted by Woudenberg (1991) as given the topic, identifying someone who is an expert on American cultural issues is ambiguous.

Later, Duffield (1993) compared the findings from two expert panels of registered nurse managers (or those involved in management education), on competencies of first-line managers. One panel was composed on 16 members and the other had 34 members. She found the two panels agreed on 93% (156 of the 168) of the competencies identified, leading claims of the reliability of an expert panel.

However, as the foundation of a Delphi relies on judgements, variances in results can be influenced by situation and personal bias (Kahneman *et al.*, 1982). In 1991, Woudenberg explored the reliability and accuracy of the Delphi by comparing the results of 14 studies, evaluating two or more Delphi's undertaken on the same subject that reported reliability coefficients (Pearson, Kappa, or rank-order coefficient) between 32 and 87. Given the flexibility of the Delphi techniques application and procedure, measuring reliability was not straightforward. Although the topic remained the same, the design (classic, modified, decision and policy), number of rounds, provision of feedback, expertise selection, composition and size varied. Indeed, studies reviewed showed many limitations, such as bias in phrasing of questions, different years of obtaining data and large or undetected error variance. Such variances were referred to as personal and situation-specific bias which he viewed as seriously hampering the evaluation to reliability and accuracy of a Delphi.

In response, Kastein *et al.* (1993) attempted to minimise the influences of situation and person-specific bias, by composing two groups of panellists under equal circumstances and in the same period of time. The two groups independently developed evaluation criteria for the performance of family physicians. The researchers attempted to control for situation-specific bias by standardising the recruitment procedure, the group size, the background information, the number of rounds, the design of the questionnaire and the contents of the first round questionnaire. In relation to personal-specific bias they sampled family physicians from eight centres for vocational training in and medical specialists from departments of internal medicine of several teaching hospitals all from the Netherlands. Each group was composed of 13 panellists, seven family physicians and six medical specialists. In Round 1, both groups received an identical list of 329 statements on the performance of family physicians consulted by patients having non-specific abdominal pain and constipation. They were instructed to respond with a yes or a no answer only. Analysis of Round 1 reported a high level of agreement between the two groups which the researchers claimed inferred a high level of reliability. However, Kastein *et al.* (1993) recognised that Delphi's vary in application, design and process therefore even 'when reliable results are encountered in a particular

Delphi application, generalizing this finding to the "ideal Delphi" is never justified' (p. 322). Leading Kastein *et al.* (1993) to conclude that reliability of each Delphi study should be evaluated separately.

Criteria to assess rigour

Rigour can be assessed by a number of approaches: firstly, by the sample number (Couper, 1984). In Delphi's the number of participants can vary from under 10 to over 1000 and as recognised the sample selected depends on the nature of the topic. Secondly, rigour can be assessed by the design selected; however, with increasing elasticity in the approach without ensuring rigour, McKenna (1994a) has warned it may threaten the approach. Finally, Sackman (1974) recommended that a Delphi study be replicated at a later time on an independent sample of panellists to enable earlier findings to be compared. However, this has been largely ignored by Delphi practitioners and when undertaken criticism has been directed at a lack of control of situation and personal variables.

Response rates as a measure of rigour

It is claimed the reliability of the Delphi is highly dependent on the panel of experts (Murry & Hammon, 1995; Beretta, 1996). However, the dependence on expert judgements has been challenged (Sackman, 1975; Woudenberg, 1991), simply because an expert panel's responses to one question can substantially differ. Indeed, some warn that group pressure results in a false consensus being reported in Delphi studies (Mullen, 2003). Moreover, Loo's (2002) claims that the use of an open-first round makes the assessment of reliability problematic.

Is the definitive answer reached?

As early as 1975, Sackman criticised the claims that the Delphi is reliable, yet in the same year Jillson (1975a, 1975b) refuted these claims, believing that establishing and application of guidelines by which the quality of the Delphi research can be tested would help ensure reliability. These guidelines include the following:

- Applicably of the method to a specific problem
- Selection of respondents and their expertise
- Design and administration of the questionnaire
- Feedback
- Consensus
- Group meeting

(*Source*: van Zolingen & Klaassen, 2003, p. 329)

The studies outlined, despite having methodological shortcomings, result in an elusive definitive statement (Crisp *et al.*, 1997). While some claim that the method is not reliable (Rowe *et al.*, 1991; Williams & Webb, 1994b; Walker & Selfe, 1996; Ayton *et al.*, 1999; Simoens, 2006), whilst others (Helmer, 1967; Reid, 1988) argued that Delphi is a valid and reliable method. With little research being undertaken in this area and the increasing flexibility of the approach, presents a considerable challenge in establishing the reliability, yet this has not undeterred researchers in its use.

Validity

Validity refers to the 'the ability of the instrument to measure the attributes of the construct under study' (DeVon *et al.*, 2007, p. 155). It is divided into external which measures the generalisability of the findings and internal which refers to the confidence we place in the cause and effect relationship, that is, is there another reason (cause) that can explain my results (effect?). There are several ways validity can be measured including content and criterion-related.

Content validity

Content validity estimates if the 'item in the tool sample the complete range of the attribute under study' (DeVon *et al.*, 2007, p. 157). For example, if a depression scale accesses the emotional impact of depression but not the behavioural aspect it can be said it lacks content validity. Face validity is related to content but does differ, as it 'means that the instrument looks, on the face of it, as if it measures the construct of interest' (De Von *et al.*, 2007, p. 157). Numerous writers claim the Delphi provides evidence of content and face validity (Goodman, 1987; Caves, 1988; Reid, 1988; Walker & Selfe, 1996; Sharkey & Sharples, 2001; Morgan *et al.*, 2007; Huang *et al.*, 2008). This belief is based on three key assumptions: firstly, the results stem from group opinion; therefore, they are more valid than a decision made by a single person; secondly, the process is based on expert opinion from the 'real world' providing confirmative judgments (Spencer-Cooke, 1989; Cross, 1999). Finally, the process of the Delphi, combining an open first qualitative round, allows experts to generate scale items and the continual succession of rounds allows the opportunity to review and judge the appropriateness of the scale. However, underlying these assumptions is the ability to demonstrate that panellists are representative of the expert group and knowledge area under study, yet are impartial to the results. A process which can be easier said than done.

Criterion-related validity

Criterion-related validity is established when a test is shown to be effective in predicting criterion or indicators of a construct. There are two different types: concurrent and predictive and the difference lies in the timing. Concurrent validity can be demonstrated when a test, administered at the same time, is correlated with a measure that has been previously validated. In contrast, predictive validity is where one measure occurs earlier and is meant to predict some later measure (McIntire & Miller, 2005). It is assumed the Delphi contributes to concurrent validity (Goodman, 1987; Caves, 1988; Sharkey & Sharples, 2001) due to the successive rounds (Hasson *et al.*, 2000) and by achieving consensus (Williams & Webb, 1994b; Streiner & Norman, 1995; Raine, 2006) as the panellists have identified and agreed the components (Williams & Webb, 1994b).

Predictive validity, on the other hand, is often measured in terms of the accuracy of the Delphi (von der Gracht, 2008) and many claim this is proof of the techniques validity (Keeney *et al.*, 2001; Okoli & Pawlowski, 2004). Since the methods inception, a number of studies have explored the short-(Dalkey, 1969a; Dalkey *et al.*, 1969, 1970; Jolson & Rossow, 1971) and long-range forecasting accuracy (Riggs, 1983; Ono & Wedemeyer, 1994). For example, Ono and Wedemeyer (1994) compared the results from a Delphi panel 16 years earlier with one undertaken in 1991, they concluded that the earlier forecasts correlated with the later assessments and that the original panel had correctly forecast nearly half the events. Whilst these findings lend support to the use of this technique in long-range forecasting, de Meyrick (2003) warned that experts normally hold positions of power and, therefore, may directly shape the results generating a 'self-fulfilling prophecy' (de Meyrick, 2003, p. 13), undermining accuracy claims.

Others have measured the accuracy and superiority of the Delphi technique with other judgement methods on the same topic. Early work (Helmer, 1963, 1964; Brown & Helmer, 1964; Dalkey, 1969b, 1969c, 1971, 1975; Rescher, 1969; Dahl, 1974; Sack, 1974; Scheive *et al.*, 1975; Penfield, 1975; Riggs, 1983) demonstrated that the Delphi method has distinct advantages over traditional group discussions, conferences, brainstorming and other interactive group processes. For example, Penfield (1975) and Sack (1974) compared the Delphi with face-to-face methods and reported that the Delphi was more accurate. Later Riggs (1983) compared the Delphi with conference groups, on the area of point spreads of college football games in advance of play. Riggs reported that the Delphi outperformed conference methods on the basis of accuracy for long-range forecasting, concluding that it offered superior accuracy. However, many of the studies in this area are dated and there has been little attention paid in this area which Ziglio (1996) referred to an 'academic silence' shrouding the debate (p. 16).

Threats to validity

There are a number of threats to establishing the external and internal validity in any study. In relation to external validity, claims of generalising may be inappropriate if your study was undertaken on a specific sample, at a certain time and place and concluded that results could be transferred to the wider context. As Delphi panels are composed of experts, who may not be typical of the general population findings, generalisability may be questioned.

Threats to internal validity include the following:

- *Selection*: a Delphi's sample may have certain features that may influence the results, for example if an expert is a patient, does the patients gender, personality, mental ability influence responses. Rowe *et al.* (1991) believed that validity is influenced by the number of experts in a sample, the level of expertise and average agreement to which experts dispose of similar or different knowledge. Sandrey and Bulger (2008) claimed that 'the results of a Delphi investigation are specific to the panel of experts. The results are not necessarily repeatable with other groups of similarly qualified members due to the considerable variation in individual backgrounds that exists' (p. 137). Indeed, as Clayton (1997) warned even the most well planned Delphi may not 'yield an exhaustive nor all-inclusive set of ideas' (Clayton, 1997, p. 382). Indeed, as the Delphi relies on the experts it raises the question, would non-experts identify the same issues? Sackman (1975) claimed that 'expert and non-expert panels give indistinguishable responses in forecasting or evaluating social phenomena' (p. 44).
- *History*: Outside events may influence expert's responses between successive rounds of a Delphi, for example new policy issued, or other research on the area reported. A discrepancy may be due to an external event occurring not accounted for in the study.
- *Situation*: This refers to all situational specifics including the Delphi design, timing, number of rounds, type of feedback provided and lack of agreement on what constitutes consensus, etc. that can potentially limit generalisability. The various adaptations of the Delphi technique have led to considerable criticism, claiming that it threatens the reliability and validity of the technique (McKenna & Keeney, 2008b).
- *Reactivity*: The lack of accountability for views expressed is also a potential threat (Simoens, 2006). Another weakness is the influence of group think leading to the bandwagon effect, influencing results. Although Delphi's are meant to be anonymous in reality, this cannot be guaranteed; therefore, some experts may be swayed by others discounting the validity of other arguments.
- *Natural loss*: The validity of the Delphi may also be affected by response rates. The successive Delphi rounds may lead to fatigue and/or dropout of participants before it is completed, consequently questioning the validity of the results (Simoens, 2006).
- *Researcher bias*: Using an open qualitative round aims to capture a large pool of items which is then reduced based on content reviews.

Rowe *et al.* (1991) believed that many Delphi studies have not considered such factors; therefore, internal validity of the Delphi is largely unknown. It is, however, unclear exactly how reliability and validity should be established in Delphi studies (Engles & Kennedy, 2007, p. 434) as each studies design; sample and consensus process adopted is unique. Stevenson (1990) claimed that Delphi findings only represent one step in knowledge and are only applicable to that moment in time and for that particular expert group (Reid, 1988). In response, some authors have suggested that additional research to validate or refine the findings should be undertaken (Van Dijk, 1990; Mitchell, 1991; van Zolingen & Klaassen, 2003; Engles & Kennedy, 2007), which may also allow for informative theories to be developed (Kennedy, 2004). In the form of face-to face meeting prior to the Delphi process (Delbecq *et al.*, 1975) or pilot study of individual interviews with members of interest groups (van Zolingen & Klaassen, 2003). For example Kennedy (2004) used narrative analysis to build upon two Delphi's she undertook in 2000, to gain a complete description of processes of care in midwifery practice. She concluded that whilst this approach had resource implications in terms of time and money, it did help to clarify and strengthen findings. However, the majority of Delphi studies rarely undertake additional research.

Given the claim that the Delphi overlaps both the positivist/quantitative and interpretative/qualitative ideals (Day & Bobeva, 2004), another approach has been to disregard the positivist standards to measure rigour, instead adopting strategies that qualitative researchers use to ensure credibility (Krefting, 1991). A number of authors (Holloway & Wheeler, 1996; Day & Bobeva, 2005) believe the term trustworthiness is more appropriate than reliability and validity to gauge the effectiveness and appropriateness of a Delphi study. Trustworthiness is composed of credibility, dependability, confirmability and transferability (Lincoln & Guba, 1985; Polit *et al.*, 2001). According to Cornick (2006), dependability refers to stability of data collected, credibility the degree to which data can be believed, confirmability conveys the neutrality; whilst transferability reports the application of the findings to other settings. Engles and Kennedy (2007) suggested credibility of a Delphi can be enhanced by the ongoing iteration and feedback given to panellists, which can be viewed as member checks and by undertaking additional research methods (van Zolingen & Klaassen, 2003). Transferability can be established through the use of verification of the applicability of Delphi findings (Powell, 2003; Kennedy, 2004), whilst confirmability can be assessed by maintaining a detailed description of the Delphi collection and analysis process. Overall Skulmoski *et al.* (2007) advocated the use of an audit trail of the key theoretical and methodological decisions made to substantiate trustworthiness in a Delphi study.

Debate over establishing the methodological rigour of the Delphi is ongoing. As there is no agreed answer, Day and Bobeva (2005) advocated the adoption of both quantitative and qualitative measurements to review the quality of Delphi findings. However, the process to achieve these measurements is unclear.

Key learning points

- Establishing the methodological rigour of the Delphi is not straight-forward.
- Epistemological debate, ongoing modifications leading to situation and person-specific bias raise many dilemmas.
- Threats to internal and external validity should be considered.
- The majority of research is outdated with most applying standards of rigour for quantitative research.
- To date, no consensus exists with regards to the correct standard of methodological rigour to apply. Moreover, no definitive evidence exists which demonstrates the reliability or validity of the technique.

Recommended further reading

Brown, B. & Helmer, O. (1964) *Improving the Reliability of Estimates Obtained from Consensus of Experts*. Document No- p2986. The RAND Corporation, Santa Monica, California.

Kastein, M.R., Jacobs, M., Van Der Hell, R.H., Luttik, K. & Touw-Otten, F.W.M.M. (1993) Delphi, the issue of reliability: a qualitative Delphi study in primary health care in the Netherlands. *Technological Forecasting and Social Change* 44, 315–323.

Ono, R. & Wedemeyer, D.J. (1994) Assessing the validity of the Delphi technique. *Futures* 26(3), 289–304.

Rowe, G., Wright, G. & Bolger, F. (1991) A re-evaluation of research and theory. *Technological Forecasting and Social Change* 39, 235–251.

Woudenberg, F. (1991) An evaluation of Delphi. *Technological Forecasting and Social Change* 40, 131–150.

8 Ethical Considerations

Introduction

The ethical considerations of using the Delphi technique have not to date been explicit in the majority of published studies. The Delphi is open to the same ethical considerations as any postal survey in that the researcher cannot be certain that the nominated individual is the person who completed the questionnaire or whether it has been the focus of discussion with other individuals (Keeney *et al.*, 2001). Modified Delphi studies also require ethical consideration with regard to the modification used which can include focus groups or one-to-one interviews. Regardless of the type of Delphi, it is also impossible to ascertain whether individuals respond with honesty or respond according to their perception of what the researcher expected. This brings us once again to anonymity. Beretta (1996) pointed to studies by Hitch and Murgatroyd (1983) who maintained telephone contact with respondents while waiting for their questionnaire to be returned. Beretta (1996) suggested that this could cause respondents to feel forced into returning the questionnaire, even though they may wish to withdraw from the study. The researcher is obliged ethically to ensure that the respondents' identities (when possible) and their attributed responses are not disclosed to any other panel member.

Ethical principles

Ethical principles serve as the foundation of ethical analysis. Each principle focuses on one goal which includes respect for human dignity, justice, beneficence, non-maleficence and the role of the researcher. Each of these issues shall now be discussed with respect to the Delphi technique which serves as a starting point for understanding the foundations of moral philosophy.

The Delphi Technique in Nursing and Health Research, First Edition, © S. Keeney, F. Hasson and H. McKenna   Published 2011 by Blackwell Publishing Ltd.

Respect for human dignity

Respect for human dignity involves the right to self-determination (Caulfield & Chapman, 2005). With regard to members of an expert panel taking part in a Delphi study, a written explanation of the study, their involvement in it, how the Delphi works and what will be expected of them is the minimum amount of information that should be provided to each panel member through the use of a Participant Information Sheet. They should be given at least 2 weeks to decide if they wish to take part in the study and to have any questions about the Delphi process answered by the researcher. Panel members can be asked to sign a consent form to take part in the study or cover letters can state that the return of the questionnaire implies consent to participate. Further written explanations need to be included with each round of the Delphi for panel members to fully understand the process.

If a modified Delphi is being used and the first round being replaced with focus groups or interviews, a written explanation of the study and the expert panel members involvement in each round of the study should be provided to potential participants when they are initially approached for their agreement to take part again through the use of a Participant Information Sheet. If they are willing to take part, they should be asked to sign a consent form, which covers their involvement in the whole study and not just the modified first round. Furthermore, verbal information about the expert panel members' involvement in all rounds of the study should be emphasised before focus groups or interviews would begin, and there should be an opportunity provided at this point for panel members to ask any outstanding questions about the study.

Justice

The principle of justice is concerned with anonymity and confidentiality. The issue of anonymity is one which poses difficulty with regard to the Delphi technique. As discussed in Chapter 1, complete anonymity cannot be guaranteed when using the Delphi Technique which is a fact that many studies do not address. This is because the researcher needs to be able to link each expert panel member with their response. The reason for this is due to the fact that the researcher will provide feedback in the form of their individual response to the previous round as well as the overall group response. Each expert panel member in a Delphi study is allocated a unique code which is recorded on any resulting Delphi round questionnaire. The data that links the expert panel member to the code should be kept on a password-protected PC and should be accessible only to the researcher working on the study. As the researcher knows the panel members and their responses; this in itself threatens true anonymity. Additionally, it is often the case that expert panel members may know each other especially in studies where the expertise in the field is limited. Reid (1988) noted that these types of smaller expert panels had a lower attrition rate than a larger panel, and she speculated if smaller panels who were more likely to know who else was in the panel communicated with each other and, therefore, felt compelled to respond to each round.

However, as expert panel members cannot attribute responses to any one expert, this goes some way to protecting their anonymity. Quasi-anonymity is the term used to describe the Delphi technique (McKenna, 1994a), and it has been likened to being in an elite 'expert' club where the membership is known but they do not meet face-to-face to discuss the issues. Anonymity has been questioned by other Delphi researchers including Sumsion (1998) and Beretta (1996). Beretta (1996) pointed to studies by Hitch and Murgatroyd (1983) who maintained telephone contact with respondents while waiting for their questionnaire to be returned. She suggested that this could cause respondents to feel forced into returning the questionnaire, even though they may wish to withdraw from the study. The researcher is obliged ethically to ensure that the respondents' identities (when possible) and their attributed responses are not disclosed to any other panel member.

Ethically, it is imperative that this issue with anonymity is disclosed to all expert panel members when they are approached to take part in the study and before they sign a consent form. The concept of quasi-anonymity must be fully explained in an understandable manner to each panel member. It is important to remember that Delphi expert panel members may be experts in their own field, but they will probably not be experts in the Delphi technique or, in many cases, in research.

In a modified Delphi technique which uses focus groups as its first round, this issue of anonymity becomes even more difficult. Morgan (1998) provided a distinction between studies that offer true anonymity and those promise to protect confidentiality. True anonymity is impossible when using focus groups but confidentiality is achievable. However, what expert panel members in a Delphi study share with others after the focus group has ended is beyond the researcher's control. Literature has suggested that facilitators share this with panel members at the start of the focus group and ask them not to share information outside the group or to discuss subsequent Delphi round responses with each other as the study progresses (Smith, 1995; Gibbs, 1997). If one-to-one interviews are used in a modified Delphi, the issue of anonymity is less of a problem, but the concept of quasi-anonymity should still be discussed with each panel members in preparation for the further Delphi rounds that they will be involved in.

All expert panel members should be assured of confidentiality from the researcher and that their name will not be attributed to any comment used in any resulting report or publication.

Principle of beneficence

The principle of beneficence requires researchers to do good; in other words, that the research or study will have some benefit to the participants and to the wider society (Weed & McKeown, 2001). Most studies, particularly within the area of nursing and health, will contribute to wider society in many different ways. For specific Delphi studies, these benefits should be communicated to expert panel members within the Participant Information Sheets distributed at the time of recruitment to the study.

Principle of non-maleficence

The principle of non-maleficence emphasises that above all else, researchers should do no harm. In relation to using focus groups or interviews, in general, Smith (1995) stated that the issues of over disclosure within focus groups or interviews can be an area of stress for participants and as such could cause them harm or distress. If using focus groups or interviews within a modified Delphi study, these issues are normally not a problem as participants are usually experts on an issue that is not usually a personal matter. However, if any situation did arise as part of a modified Delphi first round, Smith (1995) has suggested a de-briefing session at the end of the group or an informal opportunity for de-briefing where the facilitator stays after the formal focus group has ended to give participants a chance to talk 'off the record'.

The role of the researcher

Rauch (1979) stated that the role of the researcher in a Delphi study was to be objective. Furthermore, Crisp et al. (1997) viewed this objectivity in terms of three factors – methodological, that is in dealing with the feedback from the expert panel and moving forward towards consensus; pragmatic in getting a complete picture of the study; and ethical. By ethical, Crisp et al. (1997) were referring to avoiding influencing decisions. This is especially important in the classical Delphi in Round 1. During the content analysis phase of the study, the researcher must remain impartial in collapsing statements have the same meaning. Some researchers have done this by keeping the same wording as returned by all expert panel members. Discretion must be used in an ethical manner to avoid having statements in subsequent rounds which are too similar. The key here is to combine statements that have the same meaning and keeping statements separate when they mean different things even though the wording may be similar. The researcher's role is not to make judgements on what the content of subsequent Delphi rounds should be but to facilitate the process for the expert panel members.

Ethics documentation

For all studies, the process of applying for ethical approval from a Research Ethics Committee can be a daunting task. For studies, such as a Delphi study, in most cases an ethics application will have to include outlines of questionnaire from Delphi Rounds 1 and 2 and further rounds as necessary. Other paperwork required will include letters of recruitment, participant information sheets, consent forms, cover letters to expert panel members for each round, instructions to each round and drafts of reminder letters. This is by no means an exhaustive list as different Research Ethics Committees in different institutions and countries will have different requirements. Table 8.1 shows the type of information that should be included in a Participant Information Sheet for a Delphi study.

An example of a Participant Information Sheet and a Consent Form from a Delphi study undertaken by the authors is outlined in Figures 8.1 and 8.2, respectively.

Table 8.1   Information to be included in a participant information sheet for a Delphi study

1. Study title
2. Invitation to take part
3. What is the purpose of the study?
4. Why have I been chosen?
5. Do I have to take part?
6. What will happen to me if I take part?
7. What if anything goes wrong?
8. Will my taking part in the study be kept confidential?
9. What happens when the study stops?
10. Who is organising and funding the research?
11. What are the possible benefits of taking part?
12. Who has reviewed the study?
13. Who do I contact for further information?

Delphi participant information sheet

1. Study title

A study to identify research priorities for the therapy professions

2. Invitation paragraph

You are being invited to take part in a research study. Before you decide it is important for you to understand why the research is being done and what it will involve. Please read the following information carefully. Please ask us if there is anything that is not clear or if you would like more information and please take your time to decide whether you wish to join this study.

3. What is the purpose of the study?

The therapy professions (which include Chiropody/Podiatry, Dietetics, Occupational Therapy, Orthoptics, Physiotherapy and Speech and Language Therapy) constitute a growing proportion of the public health-care workforce, playing an important and very significant role in the provision of health care. The recent shift from treatment intervention which focuses on cure, to one which focuses on the quality of life outcomes and changes in the way services are delivered, has strengthened in many ways the potential role of the therapies. More than ever, there is a need to ensure that evidence is sought and applied for the effective and efficient delivery of services at both the systems and individual level. There is a need to determine research priorities for the therapy professions in the context of needs in the wider health care arena, thereby ensuring a focused, coherent and coordinated approach for future therapy research and investment and achievement of optimal outcome from all resources.

4. Why have I been chosen?

You have been asked to take part because you have been identified as an expert in this area. The research study aims to identify research priorities for Therapy services as perceived by the professions themselves, but also key stakeholders other relevant statutory, voluntary and charitable bodies and consumers.

5. Do I have to take part?

It is up to you to decide whether or not to take part and there is no obligation. If you decide to take part you will be given this information sheet to keep and you will be asked to sign a consent form. If you decide to take part, and then withdraw, you are free to withdraw at any time without giving a reason. A decision to withdraw at any time, or a decision not to take part, will not affect your employment or service provision in any way.

6. What will happen to me if I take part?

If you agree to take part in the study you will be asked in the first instance to complete a consent form and return this. This research will be carried out using the Delphi technique consisting of three questionnaires (known as rounds) aimed to achieve consensus. With your permission the questionnaires will be posted or e-mailed to you. After receipt of the enclosed consent form, you will shortly receive the first questionnaire. Simple and specific instructions will be provided for each questionnaire.

The amount of time necessary for completion of each questionnaire (or rounds) will vary with each panellist; but should range from approximately 15–30 minutes for Round 1, 10–20 minutes for Round 2, and 20–30 minutes for Round 3. There are no right or wrong answers to the questions. This study is seeking your expert opinion.

Figure 8.1   Participant information sheet

The following points are important for you to remember:

1. Your participation is entirely voluntary.
2. You may decline to withdraw from the study at any time.
3. You will remain anonymous to the other participants (or experts) throughout this Delphi study and only the researchers will be able to identify your specific answers.
4. All records are confidential. Your name will only be recorded on the consent form; it will not be recorded on the questionnaire. All information will be handled, and stored in accordance with the requirements of the Data Protection Act 1998. This information will only be available to members of the research team. All information will be destroyed 5 years after the research is complete.
5. Any information that you provide will be confidential and when the results of the study are reported, you will not be identifiable in the findings.
6. Following the study information gathered will be sent for publication in a professional journal and will also be presented at conferences. All details about people who took part in the study will be kept anonymous.
7. You will only have to complete the consent form once; return of completed Delphi rounds implies your consent to participate.

7. What if something goes wrong?

We are not aware of any complications or risks that could arise from you taking part in this study. However, if you decide to take part in the study you will be given written information detailing the names and telephone number of the organisations to contact should you have any complaints or difficulties with any aspect of the study.

8. Will my taking part in this study be kept confidential?

If you consent to take part in this study, your name will not be disclosed and would not be revealed in any reports or publications resulting from this study. Apart form your consent form, your name will not be recorded on Delphi rounds. Each participant will be allocated a unique code. You will remain anonymous to the other participants (or experts) throughout this Delphi study and only the researchers will be able to identify your specific answers. All information will be handled, and stored in accordance with the requirements of the Data Protection Act 1998. All information will be destroyed 5 years after the research is complete.

9. What happens when the research study stops?

The results of this project will be used to develop future therapy research to help improve services and individual care practices. The findings may be sent for publication in a professional journal and/or may be presented at conferences.

10. Who is organising and funding the research?

The researcher should provide details here of the funder of the research study and the name of the principal investigator.

11. What are the possible benefits of taking part?

We cannot promise the study will help you as an individual, but the information we obtain might help improve the future research direction for the therapy professions.

12. Who has reviewed the study?

The study has been approved by **insert name of Research Ethics Committee and date of approval**.

13. Further Information

If you wish to contact someone for further information regarding this study you can contact:

Insert Researcher's name and contact details

Thank you for taking time to read this information.

Figure 8.1   (*Continued*)

Consent form

Participant identification number:

Title of project: A study to identify research priorities for the therapy professions

1	I confirm that I have read and understood the information sheet dated for the above study. I have had the opportunity to consider the information, ask questions and have had these answered satisfactorily.	☐
2	I **am willing** to participate in all three rounds of the Delphi study and the follow-up stage.	☐
3	I understand that my participation is voluntary and that I am free to withdraw at any time, without giving any reason. However, I understand that the success of this study depends on all participants completing all three Delphi rounds.	☐
4	I understand that I will remain anonymous to the other participants (or experts) throughout this Delphi study and only the researchers will be able to identify my specific answers.	☐
5	I understand that the researcher will hold all information and data collected in a secure and confidential manner.	☐

_____   _____   _____

Name of Participant   Date   Signature

Not consenting

1	I am **NOT** willing to participate in this study	☐

Figure 8.2   Consent form for use in a Delphi study

> **Key learning points**
>
> ● The Delphi technique is open to the same ethical considerations as any postal survey.
> ● Modified Delphi studies must take account of the ethical considerations and implications of the method used in the modification.
> ● Written information in the form of a participant information sheet should be provided to each expert panel member at the time of recruitment to the study.
> ● Each expert panel member should sign a consent form before the beginning of the study.
> ● The Delphi cannot offer true anonymity to expert panel members. Quasi-anonymity is the term used to describe the type and extent of anonymity offered.
> ● The role of the researcher in a Delphi study is to be objective and to facilitate the Delphi process for the expert panel members.

Recommended further reading

Adler, M. & Ziglio E. (1996) *Gazing into the Oracle: The Delphi Method and Its Application to Social Policy and Public Health*. Jessica Kingsley Publishers, London.

Beretta, R. (1996) A critical review of the Delphi technique. *Nurse Researcher* 3(4), 79–89.

Crisp, J., Pelletier, D., Duffield, C., Adams, A. & Nagy, S. (1997) The Delphi method? *Nursing Research* 46, 116–118.

Funtowicz, S. & Ravetz, J. (1993). Science for the post-normal age. *Futures* 25(7), 739–755.

Hasson, F., Keeney, S. & McKenna, H. (2000) Research guidelines for the Delphi survey technique. *Journal of Advanced Nursing* 32, 1008–1015.

Rauch, W. (1979) The decision Delphi. *Technological Forecasting and Social Change* 15, 159–169.

Williams, P.L. & Webb, C. (1994) The Delphi technique: a methodological discussion. *Journal of Advanced Nursing* 19, 180–186.

9 A Classical Delphi Design Case Study

Introduction

This chapter describes a large skill-mix multi-method study that used a classical Delphi technique to explore non-midwifery duties among registered and student midwives in a large maternity hospital in the Republic of Ireland. The chapter will detail the Delphi application process and discuss issues encountered during the study. It will conclude by presenting some reflections on the lessons learned. The reader should note that the role of the midwifery assistant has expanded since this early study; this research, however, represents the first Delphi method study used to explore the role of the midwifery assistant in Ireland.

Background

Workload issues and staffing problems in health care are a repetitive worldwide phenomenon, with demand outstripping supply in developed and developing countries (Buchan, 2002). This has led to the level and quality of the patient experience being questioned (Diamond, 1998; Newman *et al.*, 2001; Gerein *et al.*, 2006). Like elsewhere, the Republic of Ireland has experienced low levels of recruitment, staff shortages and an increase in midwives workloads. As early as 1998, Bielengerg reported that Irish maternity hospitals and services were suffering crippling staff shortages which combined with increasing birth rates, resulted in a lack of qualified midwifes to meet demand. In addition, evidence indicates the ineffective use of existing professional skill, for example Stillwell and Hawley (1993) in the UK, estimated that nurses were spending as little as one-third of their time per shift on direct care duties. While in the Republic of Ireland, Ruddy *et al.*, (1997) reported that midwives were spending at least 8 hours in every 24-hour period undertaking non-midwifery duties. In response, the Irish Nurses Organisation (INO, 1999a) instructed all its members to refrain from engaging in non-nursing/midwifery

The Delphi Technique in Nursing and Health Research, First Edition, © S. Keeney, F. Hasson and H. McKenna   Published 2011 by Blackwell Publishing Ltd.

duties. Considering the economic cost of training a midwife it makes little sense for them to spend their time on activities that removes them from their area of expertise; therefore, the need to develop the role of the maternity assistant (MA) to meet present and future service need was realised.

For example, often cited as an example of high quality maternity services, the Netherlands have utilised the midwifery assistant role in the context of home births. Their remit is to support the mother, family and new infant in the early days following the birth, undertaking general household tasks, while monitoring the health of the mother and child (Wiegers, 2006). In the United Kingdom (UK), the role of MA substantially differs from the Dutch model, as they have been introduced solely to assist registered professionals in the provision of care, where clinically appropriate, in both the community and clinical settings. To date, MAs are not regulated or trained to a national standard. Throughout the National Health Service, a vast array of titles are used to refer to this role which reflects the diverse training and consequently, the variety of roles and responsibilities they undertake. The midwife retains overall accountability for the provision of care, while supervising the MAs in the delivery of such care (Royal College of Midwives, 2004), however, the tasks delegated have been determined by the midwife. In order to decide which tasks should be passed with confidence to an assistant, midwives need to consider and define their role in relation to the non-midwifery tasks they undertake.

The development of the assistants' role requires a definition of what constitutes a non-midwifery duty, and as yet no agreement exists in the literature. Therefore, articulating this is not straightforward as it is dependent upon the ideologies of the health professional. Indeed, identifying what constitutes a non-midwifery duty is complicated by the fact that many of the tasks, although not linked to direct care of the patient, are almost inseparable from it. Nursing and midwifery organisations have attempted to clarify non-nursing/midwifery duties. For example in the UK, the Royal College of Midwives (1995) refers to them as hotel and clerical duties, while the Irish Nurses Organisation (1999b) views such tasks as coming under the categories of domestic clerical, portering and catering. In response, a silk-mix study was commissioned by the Irish Department of Health and Children, to describe the work and skill mix requirements of the midwifery services at the Rotunda Maternity Hospital, Dublin. One aspect of this study aimed to define the levels of responsibility of midwifes and midwifery assistants using the classical Delphi technique approach.

Methods

The Delphi technique was used to gain the professional perspective on attitudes, needs and priorities regarding the role of a midwifery assistant within the Rotunda Maternity Hospital. The Delphi method was considered the most appropriate method to use for three key reasons. Firstly, face-to-face discussions were impractical due to time and the number involved; secondly, evidence suggests unanimity of opinion exists (Jones & Hunter, 1995), therefore anonymity must be preserved; and finally individuals who were involved represented diverse (registered versus students') backgrounds with respect to experience and/or expertise. Face-to-face meetings were, therefore, seen as impractical due to the emotive nature of the topic and restrictions on resources. The Delphi method, therefore, enabled participants to give their opinion or judgement without feeling intimidated by others. Moreover, the use of the Delphi method meant that staffs were actively involved in the research process, which was considered crucial for their later acceptance of skill-mix outcomes (McKenna, 1994a).

Initial considerations

Before commencement of the Delphi study the research team made a number of initial decisions relating to the Delphi design, level of consensus and number of rounds. Firstly, as little research has been undertaken in this area previously, the classical Delphi design was considered to be the most appropriate one to adopt. Round 1 for a classical design, begins with an open-ended set of questions, thus allowing participants complete freedom in their answers, which reduces the risk of overlooking a facet of the question under examination (Couper, 1984). The resulting opinions or judgements are stored by the researchers and distilled into categories that form the basis of the second-round questionnaire. This is distributed to the participants and, based on how others have responded, they are invited to retain or alter their original opinion or judgement. This iterative process continues for subsequent rounds until consensus is obtained.

A second issue considered was the number of rounds to employ. Since Delphi literature reports that participants can become fatigued after three rounds (Walker & Selfe, 1996), which undermines consensus obtained, this study employed a two-stage Delphi. Finally, before the commencement of the study the threshold for consensus was selected at 70%. A review of the literature indicated no standard threshold for consensus with wide ranging variances, for example Boyce et al. (1993) set consensus at 66% while McKenna (1994a) suggested 51% level. The selection of 70% was not based on any theoretical or methodological standards; instead, it was established on the fact that it was deemed a stronger cut of point for measuring the level of consensus on which task were deemed midwifery or non-midwifery.

In addition, to ensure clarity, the questionnaire was pilot-tested with midwives and students outside the research setting prior to implementation. This also helped to identify ambiguities in wording, enhance content validity and improve the feasibility and efficiency of administration.

Enhancing response rates

As the Delphi method can suffer from attrition, to enhance response rates the research team employed a variety of measures in an attempt to counteract low response rates. Firstly, two reminder letters and personal visits to wards by the researcher were employed in both rounds. Secondly, the researcher made personal visits to the wards throughout the Delphi process, to ensure that any problems were dealt with immediately and that participants could recognise and approach the researcher if required. Thirdly, ethical approval for the study was obtained from the hospital management committee and permission for access was gained from management teams throughout the maternity hospital. Finally, management communications, guest lecturers, and personal visits informed all participants about the study prior to its commencement and provided an opportunity to ask questions and inform participants about the Delphi process. These procedures were time–consuming; however, all were considered necessary to enhance response rates.

Identifying and accessing the sample

The number of participants in published Delphi studies, referred to as 'experts' varies widely between less than 22 (Carley *et al.*, 1999), to 50 (Green *et al.*, 1999) to more than 2000 (Butterworth & Bishop, 1995). However, regardless of what numbers are employed, the number must be justified and reflective of the genuine population. Following this guidance, all student midwives ($n = 79$) and qualified midwives ($n = 194$) based in all clinical settings of the hospital were asked to participate. The names and clinical location were obtained through two sampling frames: staff lists, developed by Hospital Management and Human Resources, and the School of Midwifery Student List. Questionnaires were distributed through the internal mailing system in the hospital, which helped to reduce costs.

When using the Delphi it was not possible to maintain true anonymity, since the researcher knew the origin of individual responses. Quasi-anonymity was, therefore, assured by maintaining the confidentiality of individual's opinions and by ensuring that any identifying features, such as job title and ward were omitted from the final report. It was professed that participants' responses, while not anonymous to the researchers, were anonymous to each other; however upon reflection it is clear that participants did talk among each other about the Delphi process and results.

Round 1

In Round 1, participants were asked to list eight duties they undertook which they considered to be non-midwifery. To achieve this, one simple request was circulated: 'Please list at least 8 non-midwifery tasks you carry out as part of your normal duties?' This was sent to 194 qualified midwives and 79 student midwives of which 138 (68%) and 69 (87%) completed and returned the questionnaire in Round 1, despite reminder letters, personal visits and management support being provided.

Responses in Round 1 of the Delphi were very diverse but represent the types of duties participants were expected to undertake. All participants perceived themselves as undertaking non-midwifery duties. As student midwives are not allocated specifically to one ward their responses are presented as one group. Table 9.1 outlines the quantified non-midwifery duties identified by student midwives and registered midwives by ward. It was acknowledged, however, that the opportunity of the student and/or qualified midwives to perform all of the tasks might depend on the ward or specialty in which they work.

To reduce response overlap, thematic content analysis was undertaken and discussion and agreement between the authors which helped to reduce the Round 1 response to 190 non-midwifery duties. Responses from both student and qualified midwives were categorised into five subject areas including clerical, stock, porter, domestic and other/basic care. During content analysis, the intention was to maintain an emphasis on the respondent's own experiences and wording. From the tasks identified, 45 items related to clerical duties, 24 stock, 22 porter, 40 domestic and 59 classified as other/ general care duties. These represented non-midwifery duties that both student and qualified midwives perform regularly. The top non-midwifery duty undertaken most frequently by registered midwives

Table 9.1   Round 1 quantified non-midwifery duties by ward

Ward type	No. of non-midwifery duties identified
Gynaecology	44
Pre-natal	46
Lower corridor	56
NICU	65
Top floor	59
OPD	27
Delivery suite	46
Paediatric unit	60
Theatre	29
Other midwifery services (i.e. laboratories)	22
Students	91

Table 9.2   Round 1 non-midwifery duties by ward

Ward	Duty	Round 1 percentage response
Gynaecology	Making beds	95.2%
Pre-natal	Bringing specimens to lab Filing	85.7%[a]
Lower corridor	Making beds	100%
NICU	Answering the phone Ordering stock	78.9%[a]
Top floor	Making beds	100%
Outpatients department	Filing lab reports	83.3%
Delivery suite	Answering phones	89.3%
Paediatric unit	Answering the door bell	85.7%
Theatre	Putting stores away Answering phones Washing instruments	100%[a]
Other midwifery services	Answering phones	71.4%

[a]Duties tied rank.

Table 9.3   Round 1 student's non-midwifery duties

Rank	Duty	Round 1 percentage response
1	Transferring patients	72.5%
2	Making beds	69.6%
3	Making tea and toast	65.2%
4	Delivering specimens to lab	63.8%
5	Collecting charts	50.7%

by ward area is presented in Table 9.2 and top five ranked non-midwifery duties undertaken by student midwives is outlined in Table 9.3.

Round 2

The results of Round 1 formed the basis for formulation of Round 2 questionnaires. For ease of understanding, the non-midwifery duties identified were grouped under the categories used for analysis (clerical, stock, porter, domestic and other care duties). In Round 2, duties identified from Round 1 were listed and respondents were asked to identify whether:

1. This duty could be allocated confidently to a midwifery assistant.
2. This duty should remain the responsibility of a registered midwife.

Table 9.4   Top five ranked non-midwifery duties to be delegated to a midwifery assistant

Categories	Registered midwife	Student midwife
Clerical	Make up new charts Telephone medical records, porters/kitchen and taxis Answer phones Direct visitors	Direct visitors Telephone porters/kitchen
Stock	Stock cubicles, feeds/formula, linen trays, trolleys, shower and toilet areas	
Porter	Collect store requirements	Collect store requirements Move furniture
Domestic	Make beds	Clean, wards, rooms, lockers, floors, baths, fridge
Other care duties	Collect and clear equipment Deliver messages/post to clients	Borrow equipment Collect and empty bottles Locate clients for phone calls Deliver clients post Clean, wash and distribute jugs

Applying the 70% consensus level to Round 2 responses meant that those duties that did not reach this level were categorised as 'unsure', meaning that no data were lost in analysis. In Round 2, 100 (75%) qualified midwives and 58 (84%) student midwives responded to the final Delphi questionnaire. Participants also had the option in Round 2 to add to the list of non-midwifery duties; however they preferred to stick to those already articulated in Round 1.

Frequency and descriptive statistics were applied to the data using the Statistical Package for Social Sciences (SPSS v.10). However, rather than report the similarities between the staff midwife and the student midwife, the responses have been summarised and are represented under the various categories (Tables 9.4 and 9.5).

In Round 2, it became clear that midwives and students perceived a number of non-midwifery duties differently. While they reached similar agreement on 38 tasks out of the 45 tasks listed under the category of clerical related tasks, seven tasks obtained no agreement. For example student midwives felt it appropriate for midwifery assistants to take phone message for doctors and telephone for ambulances whilst registered midwives did not. In relation to the 24 duties categorised under stock and 40 classified as domestic, there was total agreement between students and midwives on which should remain within the midwife's remit and which could be passed on to a midwifery assistant. Examples include tidying clients' immediate area, making tea and toast, and getting a glass of water

Table 9.5   Top ranked non-midwifery duties to remain within the registered professionals remit

Categories	Registered midwife	Student midwife
Clerical	Answer bleeps Ensure tests have been ordered and results received Compile weekly duty rota	Telephone for results
Stock	Reorder pharmacy supplies	Reorder pharmacy supplies
Porter	Transfer emergency clients (including babies) to departments	Transfer emergency clients (including babies) to departments
Domestic	None	None
Other care duties	Take blood Arrange scan of blood Make up medication Make up IV fluids Drug and nursing rounds	Take blood Follow up blood results Make up medication Make up IV fluids Drug and nursing rounds

for clients. With regards to 22 'portering' duties listed, midwives and students disagreed on only two: the transfer of clients to other wards, and collecting clients from reception area. While the registered midwife believed these could be passed to an assistant, the student responses revealed they were unsure if these tasks should be delegated or not. Of the

Table 9.6   Other care duties no agreement reached

Other care duties	Registered midwife	Student midwife
Accompany mothers back to wards	Pass to MA	Unsure
Accompany clients to toilets	Pass to MA	Unsure
Accompany clients and babies on discharge	Pass to MA	Unsure
Position clients on bed	Pass to MA	Unsure
Arrange scan of bloods	Remain duty of registered midwife	Unsure
Follow up blood results	Unsure	Remain duty of registered midwifery
Check maintenance of equipment	Unsure	Pass to MA
Deal with faulty equipment	Unsure	Pass to MA
Make up trouble shooting equipment	Unsure	Pass to MA
Assist clients with shows and bed baths	Pass to MA	Unsure
Answer client bells	Pass to MA	Unsure

59 non-midwifery tasks classified under the broad title of other care duties, agreement was reached between students and midwives on 48, eleven
duties did not obtain consensus (see Table 9.6).

Discussion

The findings highlight the level of consensus and disagreement into what
a sample of registered midwives and midwifery students perceive to constitute a midwifery and non-midwifery duty which could be passed to
a midwifery assistant. Results also indicate the ineffective use of registered and student midwives by the extent of non-midwifery duties they
undertake on a daily basis. Such duties detract them from their work in
providing holistic care to the mother and baby (Francomb, 1997; Ruddy
et al., 1997). Non-midwifery duties were classified under five categories,
clerical, porter, stock, domestic and other care, with all activities relating
to stock and domestic firmly viewed as part of an assistant's remit. Whilst
this study provides an insight into the tasks which could guide the development of a job description for a midwifery assistant, the level of skill and
the quality of care provided to undertake such tasks were not considered,
a key criticism of this study.

Tasks relating to the transferring of emergency clients, administrating
medications and undertaking nursing rounds were firmly viewed by all
participants within the registered midwifes scope of practice. However,
these were non-midwifery duties that were originally identified in Round
1. Opinions however varied with respect to some duties that should be
delegated to an unqualified assistant. For example while registered midwives felt physical care activities, such as 'positioning clients in bed',
'transferring well clients to other departments', and 'assisting clients with
showers and bed baths' as being appropriate to pass to an assistant, students disagreed. In addition, midwives believed that duties related to
equipment maintenance and replacement could be assigned to an assistant, whereas students were unsure. Such differences in opinion may be
explained by differences in age, experience, knowledge and skills. In addition, many of these duties may have become the routine part of practice
for a registered midwife but for a student still learning these tasks may
perceive these as extraordinary, and, therefore beyond the competence of
assistants.

To date, no definition of non-midwifery duties exists but in this study,
midwives and student midwives have created a basis for their own definition, based on their own personal ideology. The fact that many tasks did
not reach consensus among and between midwives and student midwives
highlights the difficulty of this process.

Lessons learned

Reflecting on implementing the Delphi technique to explore the topic area a number of lessons were learned. For example, this was the first time one of the authors (Hasson) used the Delphi in practice and found this to be a steep-learning curve. With no guidance in the literature to help direct a researcher in the field, decisions were made without any guidance based on experience of carrying out other data collection techniques (such as questionnaires) in other fields and topics. Secondly, the value of developing effective administration systems was not fully realised until the project started.

Thirdly, even though response mechanisms were used throughout the study the attrition rates were high, procedures for targeting those staff members on leave should have been incorporated into the study's design. Non-respondents were not followed up; therefore, their reasons for not participating cannot be fully identified. On reflection incorporating two questions for experts to complete in Round 2 may have influenced responses and therefore results.

Finally, due to limited time and resources and to avoid panel fatigue only two rounds were adopted within which no statistical feedback was given. A third round detailing individual and group feedback may have allowed respondents the opportunity to re-evaluate their own and the group's responses and produced slightly different results.

Conclusion

In conclusion, the key advantage of the Delphi technique was that it allowed the researchers to involve many more people than could conceivably meet face-to-face methods and helped to reduce to some degree peer pressure. Although complete consensus was not obtained, this study provided an insight into the duties deemed as suitable to be delegated to a midwifery assistant and those which should remain within the registered professionals scope of practice.

Acknowledgements

This project was made possible by funding provided by the Department of Health and Children, Dublin and by the participation of staff and student midwives.

Further information

Further information on this study can be obtained by contacting Felicity Hasson, Senior Lecturer, Institute of Nursing Research, University of Ulster, e-mail: f.hasson@ulster.ac.uk

Publications

Further results and background on this study can be found in the following publications:

McKenna, H. & Hasson, F. (2000) *A Review of the Midwifery Skill Mix within the Rotunda Hospital Dublin*. Centre for Nursing Research, University of Ulster, unpublished report.

McKenna, H. & Hasson, F. (2002) A study of skill mix issues in midwifery: a multi-method approach. *Journal of Advanced Nursing* 37(1), 52–61.

McKenna, H., Hasson, F. & Smith, M. (2002a) A Delphi survey of midwives and midwifery students to identify non-midwifery duties. *International Journal of Midwifery* 18, 314–322.

McKenna, H., Hasson, F. & Smith, M. (2002b) A Delphi survey of midwives and midwifery students to identify non-midwifery duties. *Midwifery* 18, 314–322.

McKenna, H., Hasson, F. & Smith, M. (2003) Training needs of midwifery assistants. *Journal of Advanced Nursing* 44(3), 308–317.

10 A Modified Delphi Case Study
Primary Care Nursing – A Study Exploring Key Issues for Future Developments

Introduction

This modified Delphi study was undertaken to explore possible developmental directions for primary care nursing in the twenty-first century. The setting for the study was two board areas in Northern Ireland (the Western Health and Social Services Board and the Southern Health and Social Services Board) and two board areas in the Republic of Ireland (North Eastern Health Board and North Western Health Board).

The rationale for this project was driven by a number of factors:

- The recent and ongoing reviews of community nursing in Northern Ireland and the Republic of Ireland
- The debate within and between the professions in Ireland and the United Kingdom on the role of the various groups of nurses and midwives working in the community and the increase in specialist roles
- The developing policy agenda around Fit for the Future, public health, community development, targeting health and social need, the Commission on Nursing Report and the support for a primary care-centred service
- The education reforms emanating from the Irish Commission on Nursing, the UK post-registration education and practice and the debate on specialist practice
- The need for a managed development agenda and informed commissioning and clinical governance strategies for primary care nursing
- The recognition that nurses make up the largest number of 'hands-on' health professionals working in the community
- A sense among community nurses that they require support and direction in a period of intense change
- The need to encourage North–South collaboration in primary care

The Delphi Technique in Nursing and Health Research, First Edition, © S. Keeney, F. Hasson and H. McKenna   Published 2011 by Blackwell Publishing Ltd.

Aims of the study

The aims of the project arose from the above rationale. They were to review the role and function of primary care services and community nursing with reference to developments in practice, education, research and policy, and to explore possible models and organisational structures for the future delivery and development of primary care nursing.

Methodology

A modified Delphi technique was used to address the aims of the study. In this study the first round of the Delphi was replaced by focus groups to elicit the opinions of the expert panel. Rounds 2 and 3 were postal questionnaire rounds as used in a classical Delphi approach.

Expert panel

The expert panel was made up of 38 primary care nurses, 14 general practitioners (GPs) and 8 public representatives.

Nurses were purposefully selected from all specialities of community nursing. Purposive sampling techniques (Parahoo, 2006) mean that respondents were selected to suit the purpose of the study and who could contribute to the discussion from their specialist background. Members of the Research Steering Group helped identify the sample. Potential participants had to meet the criteria of being a community nurse and being willing to take an active part in the project. Figure 10.1 shows the nursing specialisms that were represented.

The 14 GPs were divided equally among fundholders and non-fundholders. GPs were selected through contacts at Health and Social Services Boards and Health Boards. In Northern Ireland, GP locality chairs were asked to participate. Two GPs were from the Republic of Ireland.

Practice nurses ($n = 9$)
District nurses ($n = 4$)
Community psychiatric nurses ($n = 3$)
Community learning disability nurses ($n = 2$)
Specialist palliative care (community) ($n = 2$)
Specialist diabetes (community) ($n = 2$)
Specialist child protection (community) ($n = 1$)
Specialist challenging behaviour (community) ($n = 1$)
Specialist paediatric (community) ($n = 1$)

Health visitors ($n = 5$)
Community midwives ($n = 4$)
Public health nurses ($n = 3$)
Macmillan nurse ($n = 1$)
Treatment room nurse ($n = 1$)
Nurse practitioner ($n = 1$)

Figure 10.1   Nursing specialisms represented in the expert panel

Members of the public were recruited through Health and Social Service Councils (a government health 'watchdog' organisation). It should be stressed that those who took part were not council representatives but ordinary members of the public who were willing to participate in the study.

In its totality, the expert panel was characterised by 48 respondents from Northern Ireland and 12 respondents from the Republic of Ireland.

Round 1 – focus groups

Focus groups were organised through the local Health and Social Services Boards and Trusts in both Northern Ireland and the North Eastern and North Western Health Boards in the Republic of Ireland.

Two seminar days were arranged at two different venues convenient for the members of the expert panel. In an introductory session, a key speaker outlined the purpose of the day and the reasons for the study. Those present were allocated by discipline to different focus groups. There were two GP focus groups, two community nurses and one focus group with members of the public. The decision to separate the groups in this way was based on the possibility that some people may find other professional groups intimidating and may not be forthcoming in terms of their responses. On average, there were between six and eight individuals in each group, with each having a representative from the Republic of Ireland.

Each group had a trained moderator experienced in primary care and in group work. While the discussion was audio-taped, a note taker was also present. Verbal consent to record information was obtained from each individual. The focus groups lasted approximately 1 hour to 1 hour and 15 minutes, allowing each group to break naturally rather than imposing a time limit. The data were transcribed and inputted into NUD*IST, a computer software package for the analysis of qualitative data.

Delphi Round 2 – postal round

The analysis from the focus groups formed a template for the questionnaire used in Round 2 of the Delphi. The same expert panels who had participated in the focus groups were asked to complete the Round 2 Delphi questionnaire which was posted to them and included a stamped addressed envelope for ease of return. This approach worked well and secured a response rate of 100%.

The Round 2 Delphi questionnaire had a series of 38 statements about primary care. The expert panels were asked to indicate their response to each of these statements on a five-point scale from 'strongly agree' to 'strongly disagree'. These statements are illustrated in Figure 10.2. A space was also provided for participants to elaborate on any of the statements if they so desired. Some of the expert panels did take this opportunity, and these elaborations were explored further in Round 3, which is detailed later in this chapter.

- In the future, community nurses must work within an effective multidisciplinary team.
- Multidisciplinary teamwork among community nurses is an essential prerequisite for an effective health and social care service.
- There is great potential for role conflict among members of primary care teams.
- Greater specialisation is essential for the community nurse of the future.
- Community nurses of the future have to work closely in partnership with members of the public.
- The community nurses of the future should take the lead in the identification and assessment of needs in their local population.
- Community nurses do not have the skills to take a lead role in commissioning.
- Community nurses require training and education to take on new roles in commissioning.
- Community nurses must have equal remuneration with GPs for roles in commissioning.
- Community nurses require training and education to take on new roles in health care delivery to meet the needs of their local population.
- There is no clear understanding of the role of the community nurse among the public, GPs, social workers, physiotherapists and occupational therapists.
- In the future, community nurses should be educated with GPs, social workers, physiotherapists, occupational therapists, dieticians and dentists.
- Strong leadership is essential for the development of community nursing.
- Currently, there is strong leadership to carry nursing into the future.
- Staff recruitment and retention could inhibit the development of community nursing in the future.
- Community nurses of the future will be less involved in patient care and more involved in management.
- There is good communication between community nurses and acute hospital staff, GPs and other outside agencies.
- Community nurses must be given the opportunity to lead on clinical governance.
- Community nurses must be accountable for the quality of service they provide.
- The community nurse is ideally placed to take a lead role in public health/health promotion.
- Community health services in the North and South of Ireland must establish stronger links.
- Primary care will undertake an increasing proportion of the work done in hospital or secondary care settings.
- With increasing access to technology, the proportion of investigations and diagnostic tests within primary care will increase.
- With the increase in our understanding of genetics, primary care will play a greater role in proactive health care/medicine.
- Primary care is ideally placed to facilitate community development approaches to health and social care delivery.
- Primary care has a key role in targeting health and social need.
- Primary care is well resourced to take forward extra initiatives.

Figure 10.2   Statements included in Round 2

Consensus was set a level of 51% (McKenna, 1994a), but most statements reaching consensus did so at a much higher percentage than this.

Round 3 – postal round

The third round of the Delphi comprised a questionnaire with two sections. It was sent by post to the expert panel. The first section (Section A) included the original 38 statements from Round 2. Provided beside each statement was an indication of the overall group response to that item and the individual's own response. In other words, each participant could see how other expert panel members had responded in Round 2 and they could compare this to how they themselves had responded. Once they possessed this information, expert panel members were told that they could reconsider and alter their original response or leave it unchanged.

The second section of the Round 3 Delphi questionnaire (Section B) was composed of the qualitative elaborations made by respondents in Round 2. It was stated very clearly in the Round 3 questionnaire that this was a separate section designed to explore these issues and gain consensus on them. Figure 10.3 shows the additional statements included in Section B of the Round 3 questionnaire.

The response rate for Round 3 was 97% ($n = 58$). Of the two who failed to respond, one had changed their address and failed to provide a forwarding address and one GP was 'too busy'.

Consensus conference

As the study was approaching its conclusion, a consensus conference was organised where all those previously involved in the study were invited to participate. Presentations were made from invited speakers on relevant research and policy directives in primary care – especially those that had arisen since the study had commenced.

Some issues had remained unresolved from Round 3 of the Delphi, and in order to see if it was possible to gain consensus of opinion on these, members of the expert panel were allocated to one of six workgroups. Each workgroup was given a number of issues to discuss, and members were asked to try to reach a consensus opinion. These discussions were recorded by note takers and analysed using content analysis.

Results

Commissioning of health and social care

Consensus was gained on the following statements:

	Consensus level
Community nurses require training and education to take on new roles in commissioning	98.3%
Community nurses must have equal remuneration with GPs for roles in commissioning	84.5%

No consensus was reached on the statement 'Community nurses do not have the skills to take a lead role in commissioning'.

These findings were enhanced by the discussion that took place within the focus groups. GPs commented on nurses having key roles in commissioning and they made the following points:

- Nurses need to get their own structure correct before embracing true multidisciplinary working.
- Greater specialism in nursing has caused greater potential for role conflict.
- If 'Fit for the Future' is implemented, there will be less potential for role conflict.
- Research and evidence-based practice is essential for the future of community nursing.
- There is a risk of developing too many specialists and not enough generalist nurses.
- As yet, no profession has the skills required for commissioning in primary care.
- Clinical supervision should be introduced for primary care nurses.
- Community nursing has been a soft target in the past for reducing resources, especially staff.
- GPs and community nurses should meet to discuss primary care issues on a regular face-to-face basis.
- If nurses increase their involvement in commissioning, GPs could be squeezed out.
- Role conflict among community nurses leads to unnecessary confusion for the patient who does not know what each nurse does.
- Patients' expectations of community nursing are rising, and this puts pressure and demands on nurses.
- Multidisciplinary education will significantly improve communication within and between health professionals.
- There is a great need for nursing auxiliaries in the community.
- The different employers for practice nurses and community nurses cause tensions between them.
- The training and education required for community nurses to take on new roles are happening too slowly.
- The medical model is a good template for the development of a primary care-led model.
- There are not enough good leaders in nursing.
- Community nurses feel their loyalty is to their nurse manager rather than to their practice.
- GPs do not fully understand all the different types of community nursing services and which nurse carries out which service.
- Nurse education should not be concerned with academia but with practical nurse training.
- GPs should not be dealing with nursing homes in the community; this should become a specialist nursing role.
- There is a fear in community nursing that if you are too vocal and speak out, you will not get on.
- Members of the public feel more comfortable dealing with the community nurse than their GP.
- Members of the public prefer one type of nurse to visit them at home rather than a variety of different nurses.
- Members of the public feel more confident if they are being treated by a specialist nurse.
- The concept of the nurses' being able to prescribe medication within a GP practice is very appealing to members of the public.
- The concept of self-diagnosis from media, electronic and literature sources is popular with the public.

Figure 10.3   Qualitative statements included in Section B of Delphi Round 3

- Nurses definitely have a role in needs assessment and commissioning.
- If nurses get involved in commissioning, GPs will be pushed out.
- The nursing profession is well ahead of others with these skills at present.
- Nurses must understand that this is not a role for them.

Community nurses also offered their own perspectives on nurses having a role in commissioning:

- Whoever is fit for the job should take on the role.

- Consensus by the nurses on who should take on the role is the best way forward.
- Nurses have been keeping GPs right all along.
- Nurses are so busy on the ground that they do not have time for commissioning.
- There is confusion over primary care groups and commissioning among nurses at present.

Leadership

Consensus was gained on the statement 'Strong leadership is essential for the development of community nursing' at a consensus level of 98.3%. However, no consensus was reached on the statement 'Currently there is no leadership to carry community nursing into the future'.

Discussion points from the focus groups led to several issues being raised regarding leadership. GPs commented on their perceptions of leadership:

- GPs have a role as a leader.
- The budget holder is the leader.
- GPs are entrepreneurs.

Community nurses proffered the following views on leadership:

- The GP is the leader of the primary care team.
- Leadership skills are constituted by a good listener.
- Nurses who become leaders generally leave practice.
- There should be fast tracking of people with leadership potential.
- There is the view that nurses are told they must be managers.
- A leader naturally has leadership qualities.

Generic and specialist roles

As clearly demonstrated in the existing research literature, there are a number of specialist roles being developed within community nursing. This has led to fears from some quarters that these new roles are being formulated to the detriment of generalist roles.

Consensus was gained on all statements in this section as follows:

	Consensus level
Greater specialisation is essential for the community nurse of the future	82.7%
Increased specialisation in nursing has caused greater potential for role conflict	66.9%
There is a risk of developing too many specialists and not enough generalists	69%

In the Commission on Nursing (DHC, 1998), there was a call in the Republic of Ireland for specialist nurses. However, there was a clear directive that these should only represent key specialisms rather than every disease category. Presently, there are few specialist nurses in primary care in Ireland. However, the Irish public health nurses who took part in the study believed that their role enabled them to have an overview of the patient and family's care. This fits well with the concept of the family nurse as envisaged by the World Health Organization (Fawcett-Henessy, 1999).

Clinical governance

Clinical governance is a framework that helps all professionals to continuously improve quality and safeguard standards of care. Within this present study, the Delphi questionnaires sought agreement or disagreement from respondents on a number of statements regarding clinical governance. Their responses were as follows:

	Consensus level
Community nurses must be given the chance to lead on clinical governance	89.6%
Community nurses must be accountable for the quality of service they provide	100%

Discussion points from the focus groups led to several issues being raised regarding clinical governance. In particular, GPs raised the following points in relation to clinical governance:

- There is a feeling of becoming more personally accountable.
- Clinical practice and outcomes are highlighted.

Community nurses made the following comments:

- Most nurses are already looking at good quality practice.
- Practice audit and effectiveness are of utmost importance.
- Clinical governance is just another buzzword – nurses must be informed.

In the Republic of Ireland, the report *Shaping a Healthier Future* (DHC, 1994) identified the prerequisites for a quality health service. It was based on the principles of continuous quality improvement using tools such as audit to enhance patient care. As a result of this report, the processes that underpin clinical governance are recognisable to Irish community nurses. There is however no policy on how clinical governance will be implemented in the Republic of Ireland.

Teamwork

Consensus was reached on the following statements relating to teamwork:

	Consensus level
In the future, community nurses must work within an effective multidisciplinary team	98.3%
Multidisciplinary teamwork among community nurses is an essential prerequisite for an effective health and social care service	98.3%
There is great potential for role conflict among members of primary care teams	84.5%

Discussion points from the focus groups led to several issues being raised regarding teamwork. GPs raised the following point:

- There can be friction within the team, but GPs would like to forge stronger links in the community through nurse practitioners and practice nurses.

Community nurses made the following comments:

- There have been improvements in teamwork over the past few years.
- Discussion/communication within the team makes for easier teamwork.
- Loyalties within the team are very important.
- Weekly meetings are essential to working within a team.
- District nursing is a core structure to the team.

In relation to team conflict, community nurses commented:

- There is conflicting advice to patients from too many different nurses.
- The existing teams working in the community need to be re-thought.
- There is a need for re-training for nurses coming to work in the community.

The Irish Commission on Nursing (DHC, 1998) recognised how crucial it was that nurses worked collaboratively with colleagues from other disciplines and agencies. Most of the comments alluded to above have currency in Northern Ireland and the Republic of Ireland.

Public involvement

It was considered crucial that members of the public were involved in this research and that the study addressed issues relevant to the public's engagement with primary care services. Consensus was reached on the following statements:

	Consensus level
Community nurses of the future have to work closely in partnership with members of the public	98.3%
Members of the public feel more comfortable dealing with the community nurse than their GP	53.5%
Members of the public prefer one type of nurse to visit them at home rather than a variety of different nurses	58.7%
Members of the public feel more confident if they are being treated by a specialist nurse	53.4%
The concept of the nurses' being able to prescribe medication within a GP practice is very appealing to members of the public	51.7%

No consensus was reached on two statements:

1. There is no clear understanding of the role of the community nurses among members of the public.
2. The concept of self-diagnosis from media, electronic and literature sources is popular with the public.

Education

Community nursing is an applied academic subject that involves the study of subject-specific knowledge, skills and values, while drawing upon the analytical tools and knowledge of the health, social and human sciences. It is a moral activity that requires practitioners to make and implement difficult decisions about human situations that involve the potential for benefit or harm.

	Consensus level
In the future, community nurses should be educated with GPs	84.4%
In the future, community nurses should be educated with social workers	74.1%
In the future, community nurses should be educated with physiotherapists	72.4%
In the future, community nurses should be educated with occupational therapists	74.1%
In the future, community nurses should be educated with dieticians	72.4%

No consensus was reached on the statement 'In the future, community nurses should be educated with dentists'.

Discussion points from the focus groups led to several issues being raised regarding education.

Practical training versus academia

GP comments:

- There has to be a balance between practical training and academia.
- Nurse education courses are very academically based and not enough practically based.

Community nurse comments:

- Newly qualified nurses have the academic qualifications but little practical training.
- Grading issues are a big factor as regards practical training.

Attitudes to nurse training and education

GP comments:

- Nurses are unwilling to pass National Vocational Qualifications (NVQs) and to supervise.
- Comparability of nurse training.
- Nurse prescribing is a big issue at present.

Multidisciplinary education in nurse training

Community nurse comments:

- Lack of understanding at the basic level of the different roles.
- Education with doctors is a good idea.
- Communication training is essential.
- Post-graduate education must be multidisciplinary.
- Non-existent multidisciplinary care at present.

Public representative comments:

- The public are in favour of multidisciplinary education for nurses.
- There are major benefits to be gained for working together.
- There is a need to appreciate different roles.

In the Republic of Ireland, the Commission on Nursing Report (DHC, 1998) stressed the importance of placing nurse education under scrutiny so that future professionals are in the position to exploit opportunities for role enhancement. Particular recognition was given to multidisciplinary education and its benefits.

Communication

Most of the quality problems experienced in clinical practice can be traced to poor communications between professionals leading to poor communication with patients. Therefore, nurses, midwives and health visitors should continue to act as catalysts to the system, linking the patient with other providers and coordinating care across various interprofessional and interagency frontiers.

Consensus was reached on only one of the three statements in this section. Agreement was reached at 63.8% that 'There is good communication between community nurses and GPs'. No consensus was reached on the following statements:

- 'There is good communication between community nurses and acute hospital staff'.
- 'There is good communication between community nurses and other outside agencies'.

Focus group discussion surrounding communication highlighted three main areas.

Communication between nurses

Community nurses commented the following:

- Communication must be maintained between disciplines.
- Education of each others' role enhances communication.
- There is poor communication at present between nurses, and it must be improved.
- Regular meetings are necessary.
- Role definition would help communication enormously.

Communication between nurses and GPs

GPs suggested the following:

- Telephone communication is essential.
- Coordination of communication would help.
- There is a need for better communication and better support for the GP.

Community nurses commented the following:

- Communication would be improved through regular meetings with GPs.
- Communication between acute and community sectors is crucial to quality care.
- Joint posts would aid communication.
- Comprehensively defined roles are greatly helping communication.
- Liaison is necessary for good communication.

Conclusion

Primary care nursing is essentially about making health and social care more accessible to local communities and tackling the social and environmental problems at the root of many people's ill health and social exclusion. This report highlights the need for a coordinated approach to the development of primary care nursing, an approach that reflects health and social care policy, the emerging and extended roles of nurses and the inter-relationship between these roles and the work of other members of the primary care team.

In the next millennium, nurses, midwives and health visitors in Northern Ireland will be judged on their ability to provide sensitive, equitable and high-quality services through a range of public and private sector bodies, through strengthening voluntary and community sector infrastructures and through contributing to the development of the individual empowerment of citizens for their own health care.

Recommendations

Commissioning of health and social care

> *Nurses and midwives must be resourced to engage in local commissioning arrangements.*
>
> An education and development programme should be provided to assist nurses and other health and social service personnel to engage in the commissioning process, differentiated at the following levels:
>
> 1. General raising of awareness of the commissioning agenda and process
> 2. Participation in local commissioning groups
> 3. Full time-commissioning and public health roles
>
> *A proportion of nurses and midwives should be facilitated to gain experience and to pursue full-time careers within commissioning bodies.*

Leadership

> *In community nursing, leaders are required who are prepared to engage with individuals and organisations in a range of formal and informal situations.*
>
> Leaders must be able and willing to appraise critically and audit their own practice and that of others while supporting the development of knowledge and practice to meet standards of higher level practice.
>
> Career development opportunities should exist for those nurses who show leadership and nurse consultant potential. While adhering to equal opportunities principles, a 'fast-track' approach should be considered for future community nurse leaders.
>
> Leadership potential should be developed and resourced at all levels in community nursing.

Generic and specialist roles

Because of the dynamic nature of the health and social care system, there is a requirement to evaluate continually the balance between generic and specialist skills required for each practitioner.

Comments from public representatives highlight their desire to have contact with one main nurse who has an overview of their individual needs and those of the family. This requires one nurse to have an overview of the health and social care inputs into the patient's care, to be prepared to coordinate interventions, and to be knowledgeable about onward referral in a timely and appropriate manner. The patient's main nurse should retain continuing responsibility for the care of the patient including the evaluation of specialist nursing inputs into the care plan.

There is evidence that specialist nurses make a significant contribution to better health outcomes, reduced hospital admission and lower complication rates. Commissioners and health planners, as a matter of priority, should review current provision and establish a template for the development of specialist services to local populations.

The review suggests that communication between nurses working in the community and those in secondary care or with other agencies is not good. This requires to be addressed.

The current inconsistencies in the employment and remuneration of practice nurses compared to treatment room nurses need to be addressed. It is recommended that practice nurses are funded 100% by the Health and Personal Social Services (HPSS).

Clinical governance

Community nurses must be given the opportunity to take lead roles in clinical governance.

For most nurses a role in clinical governance will be about building upon and linking together many of the activities they are already involved in such as clinical audit, clinical supervision, evidence-based practice and continual professional development.

To participate actively in clinical governance, nurses require an explicit and systematic approach to the development of practice with clear lines of professional accountability and clinical leadership.

Teamwork

> Through quality education and experience, there is a need to develop a sound understanding of the interdisciplinary approaches to health and social welfare.
>
> Community nurses must develop the interpersonal and teamwork skills that allow for collaboration with others in service delivery and problem-solving.
>
> Nurses must work collaboratively and understand the viewpoint and experience of others while remaining aware of the limits of others' competence and of their own.
>
> For the benefit of the health and social well-being of the population, community nurses must form strategic alliances with other agencies such as housing, education, roads, voluntary agencies and the police.
>
> In the commissioning of services, specifications for service should highlight, where appropriate, the requirement for effective multiskilling and multidisciplinary teamwork.

Public involvement

> Nurses of the future have to work harder at involving the public in planning and delivering services.
>
> Community nurses must also involve users of health and social services in ways that increase the user's resources, capacity and power to influence those factors affecting their health and well-being.
>
> Nurses have special relationships with the public, and this demands a readiness to ask people about their experiences of health and how they want their care needs met.
>
> Commissioners and trusts must create a climate and culture that is responsive to public involvement, reflected in the resources, timescales, information exchange and willingness to support individual practitioners in their public engagement.
>
> Nurses at the board level should invest in developing strategies for involving the public in service planning and provision.

Education

> Community nurses should continue to share educational content with other disciplines.
>
> There are skills that are generic to the whole primary care team. These include clinical skills, communication, ethics and professional behaviour, record keeping, management techniques, patient education, public health and community development. Consideration should be given to these, being taught in a multidisciplinary programme.
>
> Integrated professional educational programmes should be established, incorporating the following principles:
>
> ● Standardised professional standards for the same clinical skill
> ● Differential standards for specialist skills
> ● Criteria for the practice of clinical skills to maintain competence
> ● Mechanisms for testing and revalidation of skills

Communication

> Communication between community nurses and GPs is perceived as being good. However, every effort must be made to ensure this is improved further.
>
> Commissioners should call for communication audits to be carried out on a regular basis in their health board area.
>
> Multidisciplinary education and public involvement in decision-making will aid greatly the establishment of robust communication networks.

Reflections on the modified Delphi

The modification of the first round in this Delphi was a series of focus groups. These focus groups were held over 2 days, and participants were invited to a buffet lunch and then the focus groups took place afterwards. The researchers believed strongly that the relationships built up with the experts through the organisation and the running of the focus groups ensured the very high response rates sustained throughout Rounds 2 and 3 of this study. Furthermore, it is interesting that the experts met together at lunch and within the focus groups during what was the first round of the Delphi. As a result they knew who else was involved in the Delphi from the outset. Rather than act as a negative force, the researchers felt that this was a positive aspect of the study and again one which may have contributed to the very high response rates across the remaining rounds. While focus groups are time-consuming and sometimes difficult to set up, in this case the extra effort was worth it in terms of continued participation and good relationships with the expert panels.

Acknowledgements

This project was commissioned by the Western and Southern Health and Social Services Boards in Northern Ireland and funded by these organisations with some financial assistance from Co-operation and Working Together (CAWT) and the North Eastern Health Board in the Republic of Ireland.

Further information

Further information on this study can be obtained by contacting Dr Sinead Keeney, Senior Lecturer, Institute of Nursing Research, University of Ulster; email: sr.keeney@ulster.ac.uk

Publications

Further results and background on this study can be found in the following publications:

McKenna, H.P. & Keeney, S. (2004) Public perceptions of, and involvement with, community nursing: an exploratory study. *Journal of Advanced Nursing* 48 (1), 17–25.

McKenna, H.P., Keeney, S. & Bradley, M. (2003) Generic and specialist nursing roles: views of community nurses, general practitioners, senior policy makers and members of the public. *Health and Social Care in the Community* 11 (6), 537–545.

McKenna, H.P., Keeney, S. & Bradley, M. (2004) The role of the community nurse in primary care led commissioning. *Primary Care Research and Development* 5, 77–86.

McKenna, H.P., Keeney, S. & Bradley, M. (2004) Leadership within community nursing in Ireland north and south: the perceptions of community nurses, GPs, policy makers and members of the public. *Journal of Nursing Management* 12, 69–76.

11 e-Delphi Case Study

Identification of Appropriate Benchmarks for Effective Primary Care Based Nursing Services for Adults with Depression: A Delphi Survey

Introduction

This e-Delphi was undertaken to identify and gain consensus on appropriate benchmarks for an effective primary care-led nursing service for adults (aged 18–64 years) with depression. Because the respondents were based across the United Kingdom, it was not possible to meet face to face in a consensus conference or to take part in nominal groups. Therefore, the e-Delphi approach was selected an appropriate and relevant research approach. As already discussed in Chapter 1, the 'e-Delphi' involves the administration of the Delphi by e-mail or through the completion of an online form (Avery *et al.*, 2005). After a comprehensive trawl of the literature and contact with authorities in the field, it appeared that there was no consensus among the experts on appropriate benchmarks for adults with depression. Therefore, while the mode of administration of this Delphi was to be electronic, the classical version of the Delphi was judged as an appropriate approach.

Sample

The first stage of the study involved setting up a panel of participants who, according to Hicks (1999), should be 'experts' in their field. Panel members were identified from an extensive review of the literature and expert databases within organisations which included the Royal Colleges of Nursing, Psychiatrists and General Practitioners. All experts who

The Delphi Technique in Nursing and Health Research, First Edition, © S. Keeney, F. Hasson and H. McKenna   Published 2011 by Blackwell Publishing Ltd.

participated in the study were willing to make a contribution and met one or more of the criteria as follows:

- Has managed primary care-based adult depression services
- Has published papers about primary care-based adult depression services
- Has conducted research or a practice development initiative into primary care-based adult depression service
- Is or has been a senior practitioner specialising in the area of primary care-based adult depression services (practice nurse/nurse practitioner, community psychiatric nurse, health visitor, GP or psychiatrist) who has been practising for 2 years or more

A total of 89 potential expert panel members were identified within the UK. This included five professional groups representing community mental health nurses (CMHNs), health visitors, practice nurses/nurse practitioners, GPs and psychiatrists. The employment levels/grades of individual members varied within each group, bringing a variety of perspectives to the study, for example practice, education and research. Sixty-seven (75%) of those contacted were willing to participate in the study. A database of the five groups was developed comprising 36 mental health nurses, 9 health visitors, 2 practice nurses/nurse practitioners, 16 GPs and 4 psychiatrists. Demographic data revealed that panel membership was predominantly male ($n = 40, 60\%$).

Setting a consensus level

For the purpose of this study, consensus on each item was equated with at least 70%. This was suggested as a strong cut-off point by Sumison (1998) and McKenna *et al.* (2002). Therefore, items rated below this level by panel members would be discarded as the rounds progressed.

Theoretical framework

In health services, benchmarks relate to the quality and safety of care. In this regard, they are similar to clinical guidelines and protocols. Practitioners and managers seek out and base their service provision around the best benchmarks of practice available. Across health and social care, quality benchmarks often provide guidance on the environment where care is taking place, the actions undertaken by practitioners to deliver care, and of course the expected end results of that care. Therefore, Donabedian's (1988) theory of structure, process and outcome was an appropriate conceptual framework to guide the study. In other words, it was expected that some of the benchmarks identified by experts would relate to the infrastructure and location of treatment and care, the procedures and processes of treatment and care, and the outcomes of such treatment and care.

Data collection and analysis

Design of instrument

The Round 1 questionnaire consisted of three sections. The first section was simply an open-ended question. This allowed respondents the freedom to identify as many benchmarks as they felt were important. It was suggested to respondents that they may wish to consider their responses around three categories (structures, processes and outcomes) based on Donabedian's (1988) model for assessment of quality of care. The second section asked for demographic information including employment and correspondence details, and the third section required participants to highlight which of the inclusion criteria they met.

Pilot study

To ensure content and face validity, the Round 1 questionnaire was pilot-tested with ten professionals from outside the research setting, including four CMHNs, two practice nurses, two health visitors and two GPs. These individuals were also presented with a list of queries relating to the questionnaire design, layout, clarity of information and content. A 100% response rate from pilot participants was achieved. In general, they felt that the questionnaire was well laid out, clear and concise. They also stated that the process allowed them to identify what they saw as relevant benchmarks and this contributed to content validity. Furthermore, because respondents would be asked to rate the same benchmarks at least twice, this contributed to their reliability. In addition, the pilot group felt that using Donabedian's three categories assisted them to focus their responses within a recognised theory, while not feeling constrained. On the basis of feedback obtained during the pilot test, minor wording and layout changes were made to the Round 1 questionnaire.

Round 1

The questionnaire was e-mailed and posted to the 67 expert panel members. The question for Round 1 was 'What are the appropriate benchmarks for an effective primary care-based nursing service for adults (18–64 years) with depression?' Panel members were given a 3-week deadline to return the completed questionnaire, and a reminder was e-mailed 1 week before the cut-off date. In addition, another reminder was sent to those who had still not responded 1 week after the deadline. This follow-up strategy for non-responders was also used in the subsequent two rounds.

Burnard and Morrison's (1994) content analysis framework was used to analyse the qualitative statements generated by this initial question. This provided a systematic approach to the measurement of the frequency, order or the intensity of occurrence of words, phrases or sentences.

Round 2

Responses from Round 1 were used to design a second questionnaire which was again e-mailed and posted to those panel members who participated in the first round. In essence, this was a series of verbatim benchmark statements from Round 1, and respondents were asked to score the importance of each on a 5-point Likert scale (1, strongly agree; 2, agree; 3, neither agree nor disagree; 4, disagree; 5, strongly disagree). As well as the above follow-up strategy for non-responders, a phone call was also made to ten panel members 2 weeks after the last reminder had been sent. This was to discuss any problems and to agree on an appropriate return date to help ensure their continued participation within the study.

The data from Round 2 responses were quantitative. Descriptive statistics were used to note consensus of 70% or greater on each benchmark. Statistical summaries – mean, median and standard deviation scores – were calculated for each item using the Statistical Package for the Social Sciences (SPSS) (Version 11.0).

Round 3

Benchmarks that did not achieve a consensus level of 70% or above were included in a third round questionnaire. The panel members who responded during Round 2 were asked to re-rate the items in the light of the overall group response using the same Likert scale from the previous round. In this round, eight panel members received a phone call 2 weeks after the last reminder had been sent, encouraging their continued participation in the study. The analysis of this round also involved quantitative data, and descriptive statistics were again used to determine which benchmarks achieved a consensus level of 70% or greater.

Ethical considerations

The autonomy of participants was central to the study, and expert panel members were informed of their right to decline to provide specific information or to terminate participation at any stage of the study without detriment. Panel members also received a confidentiality pledge to reassure them that all necessary procedures were in place to protect their privacy and identity during and after completion of the research. However, as the researcher knew the origin of individual responses, it was not possible to maintain total anonymity during the study. Nonetheless, quasi-anonymity as described by McKenna (1994a) was ensured. Keeney *et al.* (2006) asserted that because true anonymity cannot be guaranteed, this is a possible weakness in the Delphi technique. In the present study, identifying features such as job titles and areas of work were omitted from any reports or presentations emanating from the study. Although participants' identities and their responses were not anonymous to the researcher, they were anonymous to each other. Full ethical approval was obtained from the Office for Research Ethics Committee Northern Ireland (ORECNI).

Results

Round 1

The first round questionnaire yielded a 96% response rate. Unfortunately, three GPs dropped out of the study during this round due to declared heavy work commitments.

A total of 1216 diverse benchmark statements were identified from the panel. These ranged from very practical administration benchmark statements such as 'a choice of venue for appointments should be offered to clients with depression' to more strategic benchmark statements such as 'the strategic development of primary care based depression services should be multi-agency based'.

Following analysis and independent judgements from the research team to reduce response overlap, 140 benchmarks were identified under the three categories of structures $n = 76$ (54%), processes $n = 32$ (23%) and outcomes $n = 32$ (23%) for return to respondents in Round 2.

Round 2

A total of 61 questionnaires were returned in Round 2, representing a response rate of 95%. During this round, two CMHNs and one psychiatrist dropped out of the study, again due to declared workload demands.

During Round 2, 22 (16%) benchmarks achieved consensus at 70%. Table 11.1 lists the five benchmarks which achieved the highest consensus level during this round.

Table 11.1   Five benchmarks achieving the highest percentage consensus level during Round 2

Benchmarks	Consensus level (%)
1. Primary care nurses should view the provision of depression care as part of their role	86.0
2. Alternative service delivery models should be utilised by primary care nurses to support patients with depression	84.2
3. There should be adequate numbers of primary care nurses to assist in the recognition and management of depression	83.6
4. Protected time should be provided to primary care nurses to provide depression care	77.0
5. Primary care nurses should have knowledge of and be competent in a range of depression screening tools	75.4

Table 11.2 Five benchmarks achieving the highest percentage level of consensus during Round 3

Benchmarks	Consensus level (%)
1. Patients attending primary care depression services should have access to a clean, comfortable, safe environment	87.7
2. Advice and support regarding depression management should be available to primary care nurses from secondary care specialists when necessary	86.0
3. Primary care nurses should have attended at least a 1-day training course on depression	84.2
4. Protocols for the recognition, treatment, management and referral of patients with depression are used by primary care nurses	82.5
5. Primary care nurses should have knowledge of the causes, symptoms of depression and influences of co-morbidity	82.5

Round 3

A total of 58 questionnaires were returned in Round 3, representing a response rate of 95%. During this round, one CMHN, one GP and one psychiatrist dropped out of the study, again due to declared workload pressures.

Of the 118 benchmarks listed in the Round 3 questionnaire, 51 (43%) achieved consensus by panel members. This represented 35 (69%) under the category of structures, 10 (19%) under processes and 6 (12%) under outcomes. Table 11.2 demonstrates the five benchmarks with the highest percentage level of consensus achieved during Round 3.

Benchmarks achieving consensus during Rounds 2 and 3 of the study were added together to form a total of 73 benchmarks. Table 11.3 demonstrates the total consensual benchmarks achieved during the Delphi study.

Discussion

Although the Delphi expert panel consisted of mental health nurses, practice nurses/nurse practitioners, health visitors, GPs and psychiatrists, there were remarkably few contradictions among the identified

Table 11.3 Total benchmarks achieving consensus

	Achieving consensus (%)	No consensus (%)	Total (%)
Structures	45 (59)	31 (41)	76 (54)
Processes	18 (56)	14 (44)	32 (23)
Outcomes	10 (31)	22 (69)	32 (23)
Total	73 (52)	67 (48)	140 (100)

benchmarks. GPs and nurses tended to focus more on structures and processes when identifying benchmarks, whereas the main focus for psychiatrists was on outcomes. This may be because as secondary care professionals, psychiatrists have no direct influence over the structures and processes in primary care. However, as they are often involved in the shared care of patients with primary care professionals, they may be particularly interested in outcomes, which affect not only patients they are currently involved with but also patients who may be referred to them for specialist care in the future. It is also possible that psychiatrists base their definition of depression on signs and symptoms, and a measure of the success of their treatment would be a resolution or non-resolution of these in the form of outcomes. However, it is also possible that if there had been more psychiatrists participating, there may have been a greater spread of responses across the structure, process and outcome categories.

Following three rounds of the Delphi, consensus was achieved on 73 appropriate benchmarks under the categories of structures, processes and outcomes. They related to areas such as organisational structures, guidelines, staffing levels, knowledge and skills of staff and treatments provided. Significantly, the benchmarks achieving consensus kept the highest scores during the second and third rounds, indicating that although only 22 benchmarks achieved consensus during Round 2, the constancy of the responses indicates reliability regarding the results. This contradicts the view of critics of the Delphi who, according to Keeney *et al.* (2006), asserts that panel members are inclined to change their minds because of a mistaken belief that the views expressed by the majority of the panels must be right.

The agreement among the respondents across the three rounds was laudable. However, although 73 benchmarks achieved consensus, Keeney *et al.* (2001) highlighted that the existence of consensus from the Delphi process does not mean that the correct answer has been found; it merely means that, to a specific level, the participants have agreed on an issue or a set of issues.

Conclusion

Traditionally, the care of patients with depression has been hospital and secondary care focused. The current approach is to manage the majority of such individuals in primary or community care with a shared care function with secondary care for the more severe cases, following agreed guidelines and protocols defined in the National Service Framework for Mental Health (Department of Health, 1999). The new General Medical Services (GMS) contract (NHS Confederation & BMA, 2003) provides an opportunity for primary care nurses, including CMHNs, to provide effective depression services in primary care, which are guided and validated by a set of appropriate benchmarks.

The Delphi technique proved helpful in systematically identifying and gaining consensus, where none previously existed, on a core set of appropriate benchmarks from a multiprofessional panel of experts across the UK. Careful consideration was necessary in relation to understanding the Delphi process, identification of 'experts', questionnaire design, agreement on an appropriate level of consensus and the number of rounds to conduct.

The 73 benchmarks on which consensus was gained will enable primary care practitioners worldwide to identify gaps in their practice against their peers, encourage improvement in the delivery of depression care and establish 'standards' of what types of care are feasible. The benchmarks may also be used by health care employers and commissioners to monitor, evaluate and improve the quality of depression services provided in primary care. It is important that these benchmarks are linked with other research initiatives aimed at addressing the quality of primary mental health care as a whole. Although this study is an important step towards routinely measuring the quality of care provided to patients with depression in primary care, it is important that it is incorporated into a process of continuous quality improvement.

Reflections on the e-Delphi

The e-Delphi worked well in this study. The reason for this may be because most of the experts identified in the Delphi sample had easy access to e-mail and they use it as the main form of communication.

The advantages of the e-Delphi are obvious; not only is it an environmentally friendly way to carry out research, it leads to more rapid feedback to and responses from panel members. It also assists and speeds up analysis, and electronic responses can be fed into SPSS. In addition, reminder e-mails can be sent out automatically, and there is no cost in terms of postage or printing. It is also possible that an electronic questionnaire where the busy respondent sees one page at a time is perceived as being easier to commence than a full printed questionnaire.

The disadvantages include the possibility that not all Delphi experts would have an e-mail account – although this is getting less common. Furthermore, as with all questionnaires it is possible that busy people will complete the e-Delphi in a casual fashion or may decide not to participate. For some managers who may be potential Delphi experts, it is often the case that their secretaries or personal assistants have access to their e-mail accounts and this may threaten response anonymity. It is important that all e-mails are labelled as strictly private and confidential. Finally, the sensitivity of computer firewalls in some organisations may block e-Delphi questionnaires or direct them into a junk folder.

We predict that more Delphi studies specifically and survey generally will be carried out by electronic means. For example the 'Survey Monkey' is becoming increasingly popular and is replacing the postal questionnaire.

Acknowledgements

This study was funded by the Research and Development Office for Northern Ireland. The researchers and authors of this e-Delphi were Dr Carole McIlrath, Dr Sinead Keeney, Professor Hugh McKenna and Dr Derek McLaughlin, University of Ulster.

Further information

Further information on this study can be obtained by contacting Dr Sinead Keeney, Senior Lecturer, Institute of Nursing Research, University of Ulster; e-mail: sr.keeney@ulster.ac.uk

Publications

Full results for this study can be found in the paper:

McIlrath, C., Keeney, S., McKenna, H.P. & McLaughlin, D. (2009) Identification of appropriate benchmarks for effective primary care based nursing services for adults with depression: a Delphi survey. *Journal of Advanced Nursing* 66(2), 269–281.

Annotated Bibliography

Adler, M. & Ziglio, E. (1996) *Gazing into the Oracle: The Delphi Method and Its Application to Social Policy and Public Health.* Jessica Kingsley Publishers, London.

This book represents one of the earliest books focusing on the Delphi method in the fields of social policy and public health. Whilst it is directed to professionals and students within these areas, it is applicable to other fields. It provides a review of the methodological, theoretical and practical issues of the methods providing illustrative examples of its application.

Akins, R.B., Tolson, H. & Cole, B.R. (2005) Stability of response characteristics of a Delphi panel: application of bootstrap data expansion. *BMC Medical Research Methodology* 5, 37.

This paper questioned the lack of clear identification of what constitutes a sufficient number of expert panel members to ensure stability of results. Having analysed the first round of a Delphi survey with 23 experts in healthcare quality and patient safety, the authors stated that their findings showed that the response characteristics of a small expert panel in a well-defined area of knowledge are stable. Implications discussed in this paper are useful reading for the more experienced Delphi researcher.

Amos, T. & Pearse, N. (2008) Pragmatic research design: an illustration for the use of the Delphi technique. *Electronic Journal of Business Research Methods* 6(2), 95–102.

This recent manuscript outlines the practical difficulties and dilemmas faced throughout the process with reflections and lessons learnt from the practitioner viewpoint. Main Delphi technique characteristics are highlighted and arguments to adopt a constructivist paradigm are discussed. Required reading for a novice Delphi practitioner as a forewarning of the pitfalls that could be encountered.

Baker, J., Lovell, K. & Harris, N. (2006) How expert are the experts? An exploration of the concept of expert within Delphi panel techniques. *Nurse Researcher* 14(1), 59–70.

This paper explores the use of the term 'expert' in relation to the Delphi technique. It discusses the lack of definition of the term 'expert' in this context. Furthermore, it puts forward recommendations for researchers to ensure rigour when selecting 'experts' for future Delphi studies. As this is an important issue which is not widely discussed, this paper is an important paper for new and experienced Delphi researchers.

Beech, B. (1999) Go the extra mile – use the Delphi Technique. *Journal of Nursing Management* 7, 261–288.

The Delphi Technique in Nursing and Health Research, First Edition, © S. Keeney, F. Hasson and H. McKenna   Published 2011 by Blackwell Publishing Ltd.

This paper describes the Delphi technique and the potential of the approach to contribution to the management of change. The author critiques the Delphi technique and advocates its ability to produce information that would ordinarily be difficult or impossible to obtain. This is a useful paper in explaining how the technique is used in a specific context and sets out the potential advantages for use in situations where instant answers are not required.

Beech, B. (2001) The Delphi approach: recent applications in health care. *Nurse Researcher* 8(4), 38–48.

This paper considers the potential major contribution of the Delphi technique to the policy process at both a national and local scale. It presents data on the utilisation of the technique between 1995 and 2001, showing an increase in usage in nursing and health disciplines. It focuses on the repeated concerns of Delphi researchers in relation to response rates, attrition rates, the definition of experts and method of sample selection among others. It is a useful paper for Delphi researchers to consider strategies for overcoming these types of issues when using the method.

Beretta, R. (1996) A critical review of the Delphi technique. *Nurse Researcher* 3(4), 79–89.

This is a very highly cited paper which concisely discusses the usefulness of the Delphi technique for surveying informed opinion. However, Beretta pointed out the pros and cons of the technique which has been the basis of many decisions on using the technique for researchers. The paper essentially provides an overview of the Delphi technique and is useful reading for both new and experienced Delphi researchers alike.

Bowles, N. (1999) The Delphi technique. *Nursing Standard* 13(45), 32–36.

This paper reviews the use of the Delphi technique between 1981 and 1998 in nursing, medical and allied health literature. It is interesting to view the ways in which it has been used in the past and the frequency of its use. The paper also discusses many of the key issues associated with the Delphi technique. This review published in 1999 showed a decline in the use of Delphi in these disciplines. It is interesting to note that in the past decade the technique has increased rapidly in use in many disciplines including nursing and health.

Brown, B. (1968) *A Methodology Used for the Elicitation of Opinions of Experts.* Document No P-3925. The RAND Corporation, Santa Monica, California.

This early report details a description of the Delphi, problems of the method and initial and potential areas of application. A review of the modifications of the method since its inception is outlined along with identification of fields upon which the Delphi can be developed, including medical diagnosis and industrial forecasting. In addition, recognition of the potential for technology to effectively administer the method is outlined.

Brown, B., Cochran, S. & Dalkey, N. (1969) *The Delphi Method, II: Structure of Experiments.* Document No RM5957PR. The RAND Corporation, Santa Monica, California.

This report, funded by the RAND Corporation, presents evidence of early studies evaluating and refining Delphi procedures. The design and results of various experiments are reported such as a comparison of group opinion obtained from a Delphi questionnaire and a structured face-to-face discussion. A bibliography of Delphi-related experiments is outlined. Recommended reading for experienced researchers.

Couper, M.R. (1984) The Delphi technique: characteristics and sequence model. *ANS Advances in Nursing Science* 7(1), 72–77.

Couper's work presents an initial attempt to provide an overview of the sequential model of the Delphi process. A very brief discussion of the main features of the Delphi including anonymity, iteration, feedback and statistical group response is reported. Represents brief introduction material for novice researchers to the method.

Crisp, J., Pelletier, D., Duffield C., Nagy, S. & Adams, A. (1998) It's all in a name: when is a 'Delphi study' not a Delphi study? *Australian Journal of Nursing* 16(3), 32–37.

This paper discusses some of the complexities associated with the Delphi technique that are included in the literature up to the point of publication of this paper. The authors revealed that based on their explorations of the literature, rather than a simple means of obtaining the judgements of experts, modifications and adaptations over the years have dramatically changed the technique. This paper is useful for the Delphi researcher who wants to see how the technique has changed since its 'classical' form and how modifications can be used with the technique to address different research aims and objectives.

Dalkey, N. & Helmer, O. (1963) An experimental application of the Delphi method to the use of experts. *Management Science* 9(3), 458–467.

Seminal paper reporting upon the first study to employ the technique referred to as Project DELPHI. The historical value of this document cannot be underestimated and represents required reading for any Delphi practitioner outlining a description of the method, application and process adopted and a critique of the procedure outlined.

Dalkey, N., Brown, B. & Cochran, S. (1969) *The Delphi Method, III: Use of Self Ratings to Improve Group Estimates.* Document No RM6115PR. The RAND Corporation, Santa Monica, California.

This report represents one of the earliest attempts to develop and refine the Delphi expert selection process by evaluating the use of self-rating scales. Studies involving graduates self-ratings are reported concluding that such procedures may be beneficial to future studies. This report represents a required read for any practitioner adopting this approach.

Dalkey, N.C. (1967) *Delphi.* Document No P3704. The Rand Corporation, Santa Monica, California.

This report presents one of the early reports outlying the design, key characteristics and potential applications of the Delphi method. Whilst dated, many of the shortcoming and unknown elements of the technique identified are still applicable today. It presents useful background reading for experienced Delphi practitioners.

Dawson, M.D. & Brucker, P.S. (2001) The utility of the Delphi method in MFT research. *American Journal of Family Therapy* 29(2), 125–140.

This article reports on the benefits of applying the Delphi technique in the field of marriage and family therapy. A general description of the method and an illustration of its application in this field are presented. Recommendations for further use of the method are outlined in this specialist field.

Day, J. & Bobeva, M. (2005) A generic toolkit or the successful management of Delphi studies. *The Electronic Journal of Business Research Methodology* 392, 103–116.

This article reports on the novel possibility of applying the Delphi method to evaluate theory. A generic decision toolkit to aid in the management of Delphi studies is outlined along with the key stages on a study, review of critical issues and implementation factors, as well as the future development of the Delphi and toolkit.

De Meyrick, J. (2003) The Delphi method and health research. *Health Education* 103(1), 7–16.

This article presents a literature review of the Delphi technique, tracing its development from its inception to current form. Focus is placed upon the Policy Delphi and the suitability of the technique towards health education, and health promotion campaigns are discussed with recommendations to overcome methodological shortcomings outlined.

De Villiers, M.R., De Villiers, P.J.T. & Kent, A.P. (2005) The Delphi technique in health sciences education research. *Medical Teacher* 27(7), 639–643.

This paper considers the Delphi technique in the context of health sciences education research. It provides a clear and concise introduction to the technique and an overview of how the technique works. A useful read for all types of Delphi researcher whether experienced or new to using the Delphi. The authors also advocate the technique's suitability for electronic administration.

Donohoe, H.M. & Needham, R.D. (2009) Moving best practice forward: Delphi characteristics, advantages, potential problems and solutions. *International Journal of Tourism Research* 11, 415–437.

This paper presents a critical examination and a review of the Delphi technique application to tourism research. Guidance to tourism researchers is outlined.

Du Plessis, E. & Human, S.P. (2007) The art of the Delphi technique: highlighting its scientific merit. *Health SA Gesondheid* 12(4), 13–24.

This article discusses the scientific merit of the Delphi technique, illustrates an in-depth view of its definition, rationale, application, shortcomings, strengths and value. The research process is presented in discrete steps.

Duffield, C. (1993) The Delphi technique: a comparison of results obtained using two expert panels. *International Journal of Nursing Studies* 30(3), 227–237.

This paper describes a study in which two panels of experts in nursing were asked to identify the competencies expected of first-line managers using the Delphi technique. Results showed a large degree of similarity between the two-panel responses which the authors postulate may indicate the reliability of the Delphi as a technique. However, the author also stated that further work is needed in this area to confirm these types of findings. This is an interesting paper for researchers interested in the reliability of the technique.

Erffmeyer, R.C., Erffmeyer, E.S. & Lane, I.M. (1986) The Delphi technique: an empirical evaluation of the optimal number of rounds. *Group and Organization Studies* 11(1–2), 120–128.

This paper attempts to empirically establish the optimal number of Delphi rounds required to obtain stability. Based on the findings, 72 university students were initially asked to rank 15 items of equipment vital for the survival of a crew who crashed on the moon. Results indicated that stability was reached after the fourth round. Whilst the authors should be commended for providing an insight, the findings of this cannot be generalised as the number of rounds for any given Delphi is dependent on many internal and external factors.

Evans, C. (1997) The use of consensus methods and expert panels in pharmacoeconomic studies. *Pharmacoeconomics* 12(2 Pt 1), 121–129.

This article reviews the application of the Delphi technique within pharmacoeconomic research. Practical applications and methodological limitations are outlined along with recommendations for the use of the future use of the method.

Everett, A. (1993) Piercing the veil of the future: a review of the Delphi method of research *Professional Nurse* 9, 181–185.

Everett's paper provides a very useful precursor to choosing the Delphi technique as an appropriate method for a research study. It outlines various methodological approaches along a timescale which showed the Delphi technique as the main method to be used if researching or predicting the immediate or foreseeable future. The paper also provides a step-by-step process to follow if using the technical in both textual and pictorial formats. This is a very useful paper for both the new and experienced Delphi researchers.

Fink, A., Kosecoff, J., Chassin, M & Brook, R. (1984) Consensus methods: characteristics and guidelines for use. *The Australian Journal of Politics and History* 74(9), 979–983.

This article reviews the characteristics of various consensus methodologies including the Delphi method and nominal group technique. A general comparison of each method is presented along with guidelines in their application. This paper may prove beneficial to aid decision-making in the selection of the most appropriate method.

Fischer, R.G. (1978) The Delphi method: a description. *Journal of Academic Librarianship* 4(2), 64–70.

This paper made a very important point about the Delphi technique – the technique has been used not only to attempt to determine what will happen in the distant future but also to determine what should be done about immediate concerns. The paper reviewed four Delphi studies to illustrate the types of problems that can be encountered using the method. This is a useful paper for both new and experienced researchers. While it is a relatively old paper, it still poses highly relevant questions about the technique that should be considered.

Fusfeld, A.R. (1971) Research program on the management of science and technology. *The Delphi Technique: Survey and Comment*. Working Paper Massachusetts Institute of Technology, Massachusetts.

Early working paper documenting the rise and application of the Delphi in forecasting research, extensions of the method and a review of the technique is presented. Provides an insight into the initial development of the technique, case examples and recommendations for its utilisation in corporate research outlined.

Geist, M.R. (2009) Using the Delphi method to engage stakeholders: a comparison of two studies. *Evaluation and Programme Planning* 33(2), 147–154.

This paper reports the value and suitability of the Delphi method to enhancing and developing stakeholder involvement and research. Comparisons of two different Delphi formats (paper-and-pencil, postal-mail version and a web-based, real-time computer version) with two panels of stakeholders are reported. The techniques characteristics, limitations and lessons learnt are discussed.

Goodman, C.M. (1987) The Delphi technique: a critique. *Journal of Advanced Nursing* 12, 729–734.

While Goodman's article was published in 1987, it is still highly relevant to present-day Delphi studies as is provided a discussion of the techniques key characteristics which evidently have not changed. This paper is particularly useful in its discussion of the usefulness of the method in structuring group communication for the discussion of specific issues. The technique is discussed in relation to being an aid to policy, and this is very useful for researchers wishing to consider the use of a policy Delphi or a Delphi to inform policy.

Gordon, T.J. (1994) *The Delphi Method*. Futures Research Methodology. AC/UNU Millennium Project. Available online: http://www. gerencia-mento.ufba.br/Downloads/delphi%20(1).pdf [accessed 16 August 2010].

This brief report outlines the Delphi history and critical description of the method and provides examples of applications in an array of fields.

Gordon, T.J. (No date specified) *The Real-Time Delphi Method*. Excerpt from Futures Research Methodology V3.0. The Millennium Project. Available online: http://www.millennium-project.org/FRMv3_0/04-Delphi.pdf [accessed 16 August 2010].

This report focuses on the development and use of a real-time or e-Delphi. A critique of this approach along with an illustration and description of the process is presented. A case example is presented outlining the stages adopted, round format and types of data gathered. The report represents essential reading for any practitioner adopting this design in practice.

Greatorex, J. & Dexter, T (2000) An accessible analytical approach for investigating what happens between the rounds of a Delphi study. *Journal of Advanced Nursing* 32(4), 1016–1024.

This paper explores the stability of consensus and the convergence of agreement between the rounds of a Delphi study. It outlines an accessible analytical approach using graphical presentations of means and standard deviations to identify what happens between rounds. The paper used a healthcare research example to illustrate the approach. This is a useful paper for the more experienced Delphi researcher who wishes to explore the ways in which stability and convergence of agreement work within the Delphi method.

Green, B., Jones, M., Hughes, D. & Williams, A. (1999) Applying the Delphi technique in a study of GPs' information requirements. *Health and Social Care in the Community* 7(3), 198–205.

This manuscript outlines some of the practical difficulties and theoretical dilemmas faced in the operationalising of a classical Delphi in practice. It provides forewarning to inexperienced researchers on the reality, effort and practical choices faced.

Grisham, T. (2009) The Delphi technique: a method for testing complex and multifaceted topics. *International Journal of Managing Projects in Business* 2(1), 112–130.

This manuscript sets out a literature review of the Delphi approach with an example of its application in a doctoral thesis on project management. A reflection on the experience is documented along with the protocols and process adopted.

Gupta, U.G. & Clarke, R.E. (1996) Theory and applications of the Delphi technique: a bibliography (1975–1994). *Technological Forecasting and Social Change* 53, 185–211.

This article provides a review of the application of the Delphi, since its inception in the 1950s, in different domains. Analysis of the bibliography on methodology and applications over two decades is presented.

Hanafin, S. (2004) *The Delphi Technique: A Methodology to Support the Development of a National Set of Child Well-being Indicators*. The National Children's Office, Dublin.

This report presents a general overview of the technique and its application in developing indicators of child well-being. A general description of the Delphi technique, paradigmatic assumptions and pros and cons of adopting the method is outlined. Practical application of a Decision Delphi is outlined along with findings from the study contributed to the development of a National Set of Child Well-Being Indicators for Irish Children. In addition, participants' view of the Delphi technique is discussed.

Hasson, F., Keeney, S. & McKenna, H.P. (2000) Research guidelines for the Delphi technique. *Journal of Advanced Nursing* 32(4), 1008–1015.
This paper provides guidelines for using the Delphi technique and is a useful starting point for the new Delphi researcher. Many papers do not describe the workings of the technique, and this paper provides insight into the positive and negative issues concerned with the Delphi technique. The paper aims to provide an understanding of the preparation, action steps and difficulties of the technique and how to overcome them.

Helmer-Hirschberg, O. & Rescher Helmer, N.H. (1958) *On the Epistemology of the Inexact Sciences*. Document No P-1513. Rand Corporation, Santa Monica, California.
This report attempts to outline an epistemological approach to the inexact sciences through the use of methodological innovations such as expert judgements pseudo-experimentation, involving simulation processes and operational gaming. An academic definition of inexact and exact sciences is offered and the Delphi technique is mentioned.

Hill, K.Q. & Fowles, J. (1975) The methodological worth of the Delphi forecasting technique *Technological Forecasting and Social Change* 7, 179–192.
This paper focuses on the issues of reliability and validity with regard to the Delphi technique and discusses specific problems raised by applications of the technique to forecasting. While this paper was published in 1975, the issues discussed within it are still highly relevant to any present-day Delphi study and as such it is important reading. The paper also highlights reasons to continue using the Delphi technique in spite of its difficulties and also comments on alternative uses.

Holey, E.A., Feeley, J.L., Dixon, J. & Whittaker, V.J. (2007) An exploration in the use of simple statistics to measure consensus and stability in Delphi studies. *BMC Medical Research Methodology* 7, 52.
This paper discussed consensus and stability in the Delphi process and examined whether these aspects can be ascertained by the descriptive evaluation of trends in participants' views. This is a very interesting paper which will be of use to experienced Delphi researchers who wish to explore the stability of expert panel members' responses across rounds. The proposed analytical process put forward by the authors is designed to ensure maximum validity of results from Delphi studies.

Hsu, C-C. & Sandford, B. (2007) The Delphi technique: making sense of consensus. *Practical Assessment Research and Evaluation* 12(10). Available online: http://pareonline.net/getvn.asp?v=12&n=10 [accessed 18 December 2009].
This paper provides a general descriptive account of the factors to consider when designing and implementing a Delphi study. Issues such as the characteristics, process, subject, time and analysis are also outlined. Weaknesses of the approach are also included such as attrition and time-consuming nature of the method.

Hsu, C-C. & Sandford, B.A. (2007) Minimizing non-response in the Delphi process: how to respond to non-response. *Practical Assessment, Research and Evaluation* 12(17). Available online: http://pareonline.net/pdf/v12n17.pdf [accessed 11 March 2010].
This paper reports on the importance of achieving and maintaining a desirable response rate to enhance the validity of any Delphi study. Strategies to engage experts in the process are outlined as well as how to deal with non-responses. This represents a necessary paper for all Delphi practitioners to read and apply in practice.

Huckfeldt, V. & Judd, R.C. (1974) Issues in large scale Delphi studies. *Technological Forecasting and Social Change* 6, 75–88.

This paper, whilst dated, outlines the procedure in undertaking a large-scale Delphi study. It provides an insight into the practical difficulties of conducting a Delphi, namely panel fatigue, plurality and consistency and obtaining consensus.

Hung, L-H., Altschild, J.W. & Lee, Y-F. (2008) Methodological and conceptual issues confronting a cross-country Delphi study of educational program evaluation. *Evaluation and Program Planning* 31, 191–198.

This article presents an analysis of the practical lessons learnt from applying a cross-country e-Delphi study of educational programme evaluation in the Asia-Pacific region. The reality of recruiting participants, sampling, designing and implementing the study are outlined along with a methodological review.

Jairath, N. & Weinstein, J. (1994) The Delphi methodology (Part One): a useful administrative approach. *Canadian Journal of Nursing Administration* 7(3), 29–40.

This paper is specifically aimed at nurse researchers who may be interested in using the Delphi technique. However, it is a useful paper for any researcher wanting to use the method. It provides basic information on the technique including how to participate in a Delphi study and how to conduct studies using the Delphi. It includes useful information on different types of Delphi approaches and what they can be used for.

Keeney, S., Hasson, F. & McKenna, H.P. (2001) A critical review of the Delphi technique as a research methodology for nursing. *International Journal of Nursing Studies* 38, 195–200.

This paper provides a critical review of the Delphi technique. It highlights the increasing popularity of the technique and the ever-growing modifications to the technique that may lead to methodological problems. Discussion focuses on problems of definition and the advantages and disadvantages of the technique. This is a useful paper for both new Delphi researchers and those more experienced in using the technique.

Keeney, S., Hasson, F. & McKenna, H.P. (2006) Consulting the oracle: ten lessons from using the Delphi technique in nursing research. *Journal of Advanced Nursing* 53(2), 1–8.

This paper sets out ten lessons learnt by three researchers while using the Delphi technique over a 10-year period. Considering the uncertainty and confusion that still surround some of the issues with the Delphi technique, these authors attempt to share the insight gained during their studies to assist future Delphi researchers in overcoming or dealing with these issues should they arise. The authors concluded that researchers need to adapt the method to suit their needs while being aware of the issues concerning reliability, validity and ethical considerations.

Landeta, J. (2006) Current validity of the Delphi method in social sciences. *Technological Forecasting and Social Change* 73, 467–482.

This paper evaluates the methodology and presents an analysis of the application of the Delphi method in social sciences research. Explanation of lessons learnt from the practical applications in the field is also mentioned.

Lindeman, C. (1975) Delphi survey of priorities in clinical nursing research. *Nursing Research* 24(6), 434–441.

Viewed as a seminal paper in nursing literature, this author undertook a classical four-round Delphi to explore the research priorities in nursing. Early applications of the Delphi are outlined along with a brief history of the technique.

Linstone, H.A. & Turoff, M. (1975) *The Delphi Method: Techniques and Applications.* Addison Wesley, Reading, MA.

It is a seminal book on the Delphi method, presenting a detailed analysis of the Delphi technique, process, application, design, critique, and includes a detailed bibliography. The value of this book cannot be underestimated and is recommended reading for all Delphi practitioners. Digital version of this book has been created (see Turoff & Linstone 2002 – http://www.is.njit.edu/pubs/delphibook/).

McKenna, H.P. (1994) The Delphi technique: a worthwhile research approach for nursing? *Journal of Advanced Nursing* 19, 1221–1225.

This article presents a review of the application of the Delphi method within nursing research, documenting upon its raise in popularity. The pros and cons of adopting this approach are outlined along with examples of its application in nursing and health care practice.

McKenna, H.P. & Keeney, S. (2008) Delphi studies. In: *Nursing Research: Designs and Methods* (Eds, R. Watson, H.P. McKenna, S. Cowman & J. Keady). Churchill Livingstone, Edinburgh, pp. 251–260.

This chapter presents a brief introduction on the Delphi technique history, process and main features. Factors a researcher should consider at each stage are outlined. Illustrative examples of its application within nursing research are summarised and exercised to enhance learning suggested.

Mead, D. & Moseley, L. (2001) The use of the Delphi as a research approach. *Nurse Researcher* 8(4), 4–23.

This paper is an overview of the Delphi technique and other alternative types of consensus methodology. This is a very useful paper for researchers who have not used the approach before as it provides a detailed overview as well as a step-by-step guide to using the method.

Mitchell, V.W. (1991) The Delphi technique an exposition and application. *Technology Analysis and Strategic Management* 3(4), 333–358.

This article presents an analysis of the Delphi technique and a review of the applications in graduate and business research. Rationale for the adoption and modification of the technique in the field of nascent industry is outlined.

Moseley, L. & Mead, D. (2001) Considerations in using the Delphi approach: design, questions and answers. *Nurse Researcher* 8(4), 24–37.

This paper provides useful insight into the practicalities of using the Delphi technique from the experiences of its two authors. This is a very useful paper for both new and more experienced Delphi researchers and goes further than most papers in relation to not only outlining the pitfalls of the method but actually providing well-considered possible solutions to these problems.

Mullen, P. (2003) Delphi: myths and reality. *Journal of Health Organisation and Management* 17(1), 37–52.

This article provides a critique of some of the general controversies surrounding the Delphi technique such as terminology, definition of an expert and size and response rate required. It demonstrates the flexibility in application within health service research and suggests the need to avoid narrow prescriptions of the approach.

Murry, J.W. & Hammons, J.O. (1995) Delphi: a versatile methodology for conducting qualitative research. *The Review of Higher Education* 18(4), 423–436.

This article provides a description and critique of the method, its underpinning assumptions and key considerations in its application. The Delphi process and author's experience are illustrated by a national educational study which is a useful paper for an inexperienced researcher.

Normand, S-L., McNeil, B.J., Peterson, L.E. & Palmer, H. (1998) Eliciting expert opinion using the Delphi technique: identifying performance indicators for cardiovascular disease. *International Society for Quality in Health Care* 10, 247–260.

This paper reports on the process of eliciting and integrating five diverse expert panels in a national study to establish performance measures. It provides guidance on how to combine expert opinion and identifies sources of variability and statistical analysis. Required reading for any researcher complementing undertaking a Delphi on distinct expert groups.

Novakowski, N. & Wellar, B. (2008) Using the Delphi technique in normative planning research: methodological design considerations. *Environmental and Planning A* 40, 1485–1500.

This manuscript advocates the adoption of the Delphi technique in urban, regional and ecosystem planning research. Historical roots of the techniques are outlined along with different designs, relevance and transparency of designs. Flowchart of the normative design is outlined with each stage explained. It provides informative background reading on the breakdown of the Delphi process.

Okoli, C. & Pawlowski, S.D. (2004) The Delphi method as a research tool: an example, design considerations and applications. *Information and Management* 42, 15–29.

This paper presents a critical review of the applications of the Delphi technique in the field of information system research to aid management decision-making. Sloppy execution of the approach is acknowledged with recommendations on the selection of experts and design choices outlined. An example of the application of the method to identify key factors affecting the diffusion of e-commerce is illustrated.

Ono, R. & Wedemeyer, D.J. (1994) Assessing the validity of the Delphi technique. *Futures* 62(3,) 982–403.

This paper reports upon seminal research exploring the validity of forecasting trends from early Delphi study in the field of communication. Although the reliability of the method has been refuted, this paper presents evidence of the long-range forecasting accuracy of the method.

Powell, C. (2003) The Delphi technique: myths and realities. *Journal of Advanced Nursing* 41(4), 376–382.

This paper provides a methodological overview of the Delphi technique, outlining the key concept and principles. The author concluded that the technique should be used with caution, but that it appears to be an established method of harnessing the opinions of diverse groups of experts on specific problems. A useful paper for revision of the key characteristics of the technique.

Rauch, W. (1979) The Decision Delphi. *Technological Forecasting and Social Change* 15, 159–169.

Seminal paper, reporting upon the origin and design of the decision Delphi used to make decisions on social developments. Practical applications of the decision Delphi are provided along with comparisons between classical, policy and decision designs. A necessary read for any researcher implementing this form of design in practice.

Rayens, M.K. & Hahn, E.J. (2000) Building consensus using the policy Delphi method. *Policy, Politics and Nursing Practice* 1(4), 308–315.

This paper describes the application of a policy Delphi method in establishing consensus for public policy. Application of a two-round Delphi is illustrated along with the choice of using the interquartile deviation to measure consensus and McNemar's test to quantify the degree of shift in responses between the stages.

Rieger, W.G. (1986) Directions in Delphi developments: dissertations and their quality. *Technological Forecasting and Social Change* 29, 195–204.

This article presents a review of the development and application of the Delphi technique in dissertations. Over time the several stages of the Delphi's expansion are outlined with examples cited. Trends in the execution of Delphi method across various research fields are outlined as well as recommendations for the need for quality control measures are to be implemented.

Riggs, W.E. (1983) The Delphi technique an experimental evaluation. *Technological Forecasting and Social Change* 23, 89–94.

The issue of Delphi forecasting accuracy is explored within this paper. A review of the previous research is outlined highlighting little substantive work on the area. Experiment using college students, comparing the accuracy of long-range forecasts using the Delphi and the conference method are reported.

Rowe, G., Wright, G. & Bloger, F. (1991) Delphi: a reevaluation of research and theory. *Technological Forecasting and Social Change* 39, 235–251.

This paper presents a critical review of the Delphi technique with respect to ameliorating process loss. Issues of generalisability as well as the theory underpinning the Delphi process are discussed.

Rowe, G., Wright, G. & McColl, A. (2005) Judgement change during Delphi-like procedures: the role of majority influence, expertise and confidence. *Technological Forecasting and Change* 72, 377–399.

This paper explored individual opinion change and judgemental accuracy in Delphi-type studies. This paper would be of interest to the more experienced Delphi researcher who is interested in the impact of feedback and the way in which this feedback is given to expert panel members. The paper stated that the majority opinion exerts strong influence on minority opinion. It described the implications of this in relation to the conduct of the Delphi, particularly when choosing a method of feedback between each round.

Sackman, H. (1975) *Delphi Critique: Expert Opinions, Forecasting, and Group Process*. DC Heath, Lexington, Massachusetts.

Funded by the RAND Corporation, this report represents one of the earliest critiques of the use of the Delphi method. Presenting scientific arguments such as the lack of adherence to psychometric standards and the indiscriminate execution of Delphi studies were used to challenge the use of the method.

Shields, T.J., Silcock, G.W.H., Donegan, H.A. & Bell, Y.A. (1987) Methodological problems associated with the use of the Delphi technique. *Fire Technology* 23(3), 175–185.

Shields and colleagues examine the methodological shortcomings of the technique with respect to its development and application in fire safety evaluations. It explores the decision-making process of experts versus non-experts and the impact upon responses. This paper provides a good overview towards the main problems of a Delphi such as questionnaire design, definition for key terms and establishing reliability and validity.

Simoens, S. (2006) Using the Delphi technique in economic evaluation: time to revisit the oracle? *Journal of Clinical Pharmacy and Therapeutics* 31, 519–522.
This paper reports upon the feasibility of the Delphi method in economic evaluation research. The current use of the method in this field is reviewed along with several suggestions to improve its application.

Sitt-Gohdes, W.L. & Crews, T.B. (2004) The Delphi technique: a research strategy for career and technical education. *Journal of Career and technical Education* 20(2), 55–67.
The authors provide a rational for the adoption of the Delphi technique within the field of career and technical education research. Strengths and weaknesses of the approach are discussed, along with the uses, stages and the attainment of consensus. Illustrated throughout with examples.

Skulmoski, G.J., Hartman, F.T. & Krahn, J. (2007) The Delphi method for graduate research. *Journal of Information Technology Education* 6. Available online: http://informingscience.org/jite/documents/Vol6/JITEv6p001-021Skulmoski212.pdf [accessed 9 Feb 2010].
This piece of writing reviews and summarises the application of Delphi designs in non-information systems, information systems and graduate research. The evolution of the classical Delphi and its wider application in information system research are presented. Reflections from the field are presented which may prove useful for inexperienced researchers.

Stewart, T.R. (1987) The Delphi technique and judgemental forecasting. *Climatic Change* 11, 97–113.
This paper presents the controversy surrounding the use of the Delphi technique with regards to controlling psychological effects and measuring reliability and validity. A multimethod approach to evaluating judgemental forecasting is proposed.

Strauss, H.J. & Ziegler, L.H. (1975) The Delphi technique: an adaptive research tool. *British Journal of Occupational Therapy* 61(4), 153–156.
While this paper is over 30 years old, it is still a very highly cited paper and well worth reading for new and experienced Delphi researchers. It provides an interesting overview and background to the origins of the technique and a detailed list of the key characteristics of the method. The different types of Delphi utilised at the time of publication are also described.

Sumsion, T. (1998) The Delphi technique: an adaptive research tool. *British Journal of Occupational Therapy* 61(4), 153–156.
This paper aimed to introduce the technique to occupational therapists that may be searching for a user-friendly method of undertaking research. The paper explained the technique in a simple way, making it useful for the new Delphi researcher to understand. It discussed the key elements of the Delphi and the advantages and disadvantages of using the method. The application of the technique to rehabilitation and management is also discussed, making it particularly useful reading for allied health researchers.

Von der Gracht, H.A. (2008) *The Future of Logistics: Scenarios for 2025.* Gabler edition Wissenschaft, Germany.
This report presents the findings of a two-round modified Delphi with 30 logistics specialists regarding scenario planning. The findings will aid the planning development for long-term logistics decisions. A critical review of the technique based on international sources is presented.

Walker, A.M. & Selfe, J. (1996) The Delphi method: a useful tool for the allied health researcher. *British Journal of Therapy and Rehabilitation* 3(12), 677–681.
This paper provided a critical review of the Delphi technique which included a tabular view of all the adaptation of the classical Delphi approach. It also puts forward a series of questions that the researcher should consider when using the Delphi technique, and this is particularly useful for the new Delphi researcher. The paper considered the use of each round and the statistics and feedback to be given to the expert panel. It is interesting to see the types of Delphi studies that have been undertaken in allied health and to note Walker and Selfe's suggestions for its use in the field of paramedic research.

Williams, P.L. & Webb, C. (1994) The Delphi technique: An adaptive research tool. *British Journal of Occupational Therapy* 61(4) 153–156.
This paper discusses the Delphi technique in relation to nursing studies as it is increasingly being used in this discipline. The authors explore the important issues of consensus, validity and reliability and make recommendations for improving these aspects of the technique in future studies. This is a useful paper for both new and experienced Delphi researchers with particular focus on three of the most important aspects of the technique. It will provide insight into different views on these aspects and how to maximise getting the best from the technique.

Woudenberg, F. (1991) An evaluation of Delphi. *Technological Forecasting and Social Change* 40, 131–150.
Seminal paper reviewing early studies exploring the accuracy and reliability of the Delphi technique. It reports that no evidence exists which can support the accuracy of the approach over other judgement and/or consensus methods. Instead, consensus is influenced by group pressure via statistical feedback to participants.

Yousuf, M I. (2007) Using expert's opinions through Delphi technique. *Practical Assessment, Research and Evaluation* 12(4), 1–8.
This paper outlines the essential components of the Delphi process, areas of application and variants of the method. Basic steps of the Delphi process including a review of the limitations, strengths and appropriateness of the methods and how consensus is obtained are discussed.

References

Adler, M. & Ziglio, E. (1996) *Gazing into the Oracle: The Delphi Method and its Application to Social Policy and Public Health*. Jessica Kingsley Publishers, London.

Aichholzer, G. (2001) The Austrian foresight programme: organization and expert profile. *International Journal of Technology Management* 21(7/8), 739–755.

Akins, R., Tolson, H. & Cole, B.R. (2005) Stability of response characteristics of a Delphi panel: application of bootstrap data expansion. *BMC Medical Research Methodology 5, 37*. Available online: http://www.biomedcentral.com/1471-2288/5/37 [accessed 2 February 2010].

Alahlafi, A. & Burge, S. (2005) What should undergraduet medical students know about proriasis? Involving patients in curriculum development: modified Delphi technique. *British Medical Journal* 330, 633–636.

Albrecht, M.N. & Perry, K.M. (1992) Home health care. Delineation of research priorities and formation of a national network group. *Clinical Nursing Research* 1, 305–311.

Alderson, C, Gallimore, I. & Gorman, R. (1992) Research priorities of VA nurses: a Delphi study. *Military Medicine* 157, 462–465.

Alexander, J. & Kroposki, M. (1999) Outcomes for community health practice. *Journal of Nursing Administration* 29, 49–56.

Alexandrov, A.V., Pullicino, P.M., Meslin, E.M. & Norris, J.W. (1996) Agreement on disease-specific criteria for do-not-resuscitate orders in acute stroke. *Stroke* 27, 232–237.

Altheide, D. & Johnson, J. (1994) Criteria for assessing interpretive validity in qualitative research. In: *Handbook of Qualitative Research* (Eds, N.K. Denzin & Y.S. Lincoln). Sage Publications, London, pp. 485–499.

Ament, R.H. (1970) Comparison of Delphi forecasting studies in 1964 and 1969. *Futures* 1, 35–44.

Amos, T. & Pearse, N. (2008) Pragmatic research design: an illustration of the use of the Delphi technique. *The Electronic Journal of Business Research Methods* 6(2), 95–102.

Andronovich, G. (1995) *Developing Community Participation and Consensus: the Delphi Technique Community Ventures*. Western Regional Extension Publication, Los Angeles, California.

Annells, M., Averis, A., Brown, J., Gardner, A., Hockley, C., Surguy, S. & Thornton, D. (1997) *An Inquiry of Research Priorities in Nursing and Midwifery in South Australia Using a Delphi Technique*. Australian Institute of Nursing Research, Adelaide. Available online: http://www.ncbi.nlm.nih.gov/pmc/articles/PMC1318466/ [accessed 14 November 2009].

Annells, M., DeRoche, M., Koch, T., Lewin, G. & Lucke, J. (2005) A Delphi study of district nursing research priorities in Australia. *Applied Nursing Research* 18(1), 36–43.

Applund, B. (1966) The nurse's role tomorrow. *International Nursing Review* 13(Nov/ Dec), 25–33.

Avery, A., Savelyich, B., Sheikh, A., Cantrill, J., Morris, C.J., Fernando, B., Bainbridge, M., Horsfield, P. & Teasdale, S. (2005) Identifying and establishing consensus on the most important safety features of GP computer systems: e-Delphi study. *Informatics in Primary Care* 13(1), 3–11.

Ayton, P. (1992) On the competence and incompetence of experts. In: *Expertise and Decision Support* (Eds G. Wright & F. Bolger). Plenum Press, London, pp. 77–105.

Ayton, P., Ferrell, W.R. & Stewart, T.R. (1999) Commentaries on 'The Delphi technique as a forecasting tool: issues and analysis' by Rowe and Wright. *International Journal of Forecasting* 15, 377–381.

Bäck-Pettersson, S., Hermansson, E., Sernert, N. & Björkelund, C. (2008) Research priorities in nursing – a Delphi study among Swedish nurses. *Journal of Clinical Nursing* 17(16), 2221–2231.

Baker, J., Lovell, K. & Harris, N. (2006) How expert are the experts? An exploration of the concept of 'expert' within Delphi panel techniques. *Nurse Researcher* 14(1), 59–70.

Bardecki, M.J. (1984) Participants' responses to the Delphi method: an attitudinal perspective. *Technological Forecasting and Social Change* 5, 281–292.

Barnette, J., Danielson, L.C. & Algozzine, R.F. (1978) Delphi methodology: an empirical investigation. *Educational Research Quarterly* 3(1), 67–73.

Barrett, S., Kristjanson, L.J., Sinclair, T. & Hyde, S. (2001) Priorities for adult cancer nursing research: a West Australian replication. *Cancer Nursing* 24(2), 88–98.

Bartu, A., Nelson, M., Christine, N.G., McGowan, S. & Robertson J. (1991) A Delphi survey of clinical nursing research priorities in Western Australia. *The Australian Journal of Advanced Nursing* 8, 29–33.

Bartu, A., Mcgowan, S., Nelson, M., Ng, C. & Robertson, B. (1993) A Western Australian Delphi survey of staff development research priorities. *Journal of Nursing Staff Development* 9(3), 141–147.

Bayley, E.W., Richmond, T., Noroian, E.L. & Allen, L.R. (1994) A Delphi study on research priorities for trauma nursing. *American Journal of Critical Care* 3(3), 208–216.

Bayley, E.W., MacLean, S.L., Desy, P., McMahon, M. & Broomall, C.E.N. (2004) ENA's Delphi study on national research priorities for emergency nurses in the United States. *Journal of Emergency Nursing* 30(1), 12–21.

Beattie, A., Hek, G., Ross, K. & Galvin, K. (2004) Future career pathways in nursing and midwifery. A Delphi survey of nurses and midwives in South West England. *NT Research* 9(5), 348–364.

Becker, G.E. & Roberts, T. (2009) Do we agree? Using a Delphi technique to develop consensus on skills of hand expression. *Journal of Human Lactation* 25(2), 220–225.

Bedford, M.T. (1972) *The Value of Competing Panels of Experts and the Impact of 'Drop-Outs' on Delphi Results. Delphi: The Bell Canada Experience*. Bell Corporation, Montreal.

Beech, B.F. (1991) Changes: the Delphi technique adapted for classroom evaluation of clinical placements. *Nurse Education Today* 11, 207–212.

Beech, B.F. (1997) Studying the future: a Delphi survey of how multidisciplinary clinical staffs view the likely development of two community mental health centres over the course of the next two years. *Journal of Advanced Nursing* 25, 331–338.

Beech, B. (1999) Go the extra mile-use the Delphi Technique. *Journal of Nursing Management* 7(5), 281–288.

Bell, P., Daly, J. & Chang, E. (1997) A study of the educational and research priorities of registered nurses in rural Australia. *Journal of Advanced Nursing* 25(4), 794–800.

Bender, D.A., Strack, A.E., Ebright, G.W. & Von Haunalter, G. (1969) Delphic study examines developments in medicine. *Futures* 1(4), 289–303.

Beretta, R. (1996) A critical review of the Delphi Technique. *Nurse Researcher* 3(4), 79–89.

Bielenberg, K. (1998) Don't have your baby on a Tuesday. *Irish Independent* 15, 15.

Binkley, J., Finch, E., Hall, J., Black, T. & Gowland, C. (1993) Diagnostic classification of patients with low back pain: report on a survey of physical therapy experts. *Physical Therapy* 73, 138–155.

Biondo, P., Nekolaichuk, C., Stiles, C., Fainsinger, R. & Hagen, N. (2008) Applying the Delphi process to palliative care tool development: lessons learned. *Support Care Cancer* 16, 935–942.

Blackburn, S. (1999) *Think*. Oxford University Press, Oxford.

Blass, E. (2003) Researching the future: method or madness? *Futures* 35(10), 1041–1054.

Bond, S. & Bond, J. (1982) A Delphi survey of clinical nursing research priorities. *Journal of Advanced Nursing* 7(6), 565–567.

Bork, C.E. (1993) *Research in Physical Therapy*. J.B, Lippincott Co, Philadelphia.

Bowles, N. (1999) The Delphi technique. *Nursing Standard* 13(45), 32–36.

Bowling, A. (1997) *Research Methods in Health: Investigating Health and Health Services*. Open University Press, Buckingham.

Boyce, W., Gowland, C., Russell, D., Goldsmith, C., Rosenbaum, P., Plews, N. & Lane, M. (1993) Consensus methodology in the development and content validation of a gross performance measure. *Physiotherapy Canada* 45(2), 94–100.

Bramwell, L. & Hykawy, E. (1974) The Delphi technique: a possible tool for predicting future events in nursing education. *Nursing Papers (Canada)* 69(1), 23–32.

Brender, J., Nohr, C. & McNair, P. (2000) Research needs and priorities in health informatics. *International Journal of Medical Informatics* 58–59(1), 257–289.

Briedenhann J. & Butts S. (2006) The application of the Delphi technique to rural tourism project evaluation. *Current Issues in Tourism* 9(2), 171–190.

Brockhaus, W.L. & Michelsen, J.F. (1977) An analysis of prior Delphi applications and some observations on its future applicability. *Technological Forecasting and Social Change* 10, 103–110.

Brooks, K.W. (1979) Delphi technique; expanding applications. *North Central Association Quarterly* 53(3), 377–385.

Brooks, N. & Barrett, A. (2003) Identifying nurse and health visitor priorities in a PCT using the Delphi technique. *British Journal of Community Nursing* 8(8), 376–80.

Broome, M.E., Woodring, B. & O'Connor-Von, S. (1996) Research priorities for the nursing of children and their families: a study. *Journal of Pediatric Nursing* 11(5), 281–287.

Brown, B. (1968) *Delphi Process: A Methodology Used for the Elicitation of Opinions of Experts*. Document No P3925, The RAND Corporation, Santa Monica, California.

Brown, B. & Helmer, O. (1964) *Improving the Reliability of Estimates Obtained from a Consensus of Experts*. Document No P2986, The RAND Corporation, Santa Monica, California.

Browne, N., Robinson, L. & Richardson, A. (2002) A Delphi study on the research priorities of European Oncology nurses. *European Journal of Oncology Nursing* 6(3), 133–144.

Buchan, J. (2002) Global nursing shortages. *British Medical Journal* 324(7340), 751–752.

Buck, A.J., Gross, M., Hakim, S. & Weinblatt, J. (1993) Using the Delphi process to analyse social policy implementation – a post hoc case from vocational rehabilitation. *Policy Sciences* 26(4), 271–288.

Burgess, R.G. (1984) *In the Field: An Introduction to Field Research*. Unwin Hyman, London.

Burgess, H. & Spangler, B. (2003) Consensus building. In: *Beyond Intractability* (Eds, G. Burgess & H. Burgess). Conflict Research Consortium, University of Colorado, Boulder.

Burnard, P. (1991) A method of analysing interview transcripts in qualitative research. *Nurse Education Today* 11(6), 461–466.

Burnard, P. & Morrison, P. (1994) *Nursing Research in Action: Developing Basic Skills*. Macmillan Press Limited, London.

Burns, F.M. (1998) Essential components of schizophrenia care: a Delphi approach. *Acta Psychiatry Scand* 98, 400–405.

Burnside, H. & Lenburg, C.E. (1970) Nursing in the decade ahead. *American Journal of Nursing* 70(10), 2118–2119.

Butler, M.M., Meehan, T.C., Kemple, M., Drennan, J., Treacy, M. & Johnson, M. (2009) Identifying research priorities for midwifery in Ireland. *Midwifery* 25(5), 576–587.

Butterworth, T. & Bishop, V. (1995) Identifying the characteristics of optimum practice: findings from a survey of practice experts in nursing, midwifery and health visiting. *Journal of Advanced Nursing* 22, 24–32.

Byrne, S., Wake, M., Blumberg, D. & Dibley, M. (2008) Identifying priority areas for longitudinal research in childhood obesity: Delphi technique survey. *International Journal of Pediatric Obesity* 3(2), 120–122.

Cantrill, J.A., Sibbald, B. & Buetow, S. (1996) The Delphi and nominal group techniques in health services research. *International Journal of Pharmacy Practice* 4(2), 67–74.

Carley, S., Mackway-Jones, K. & Donnan, S. (1999) Delphi study into planning for care of children in major incidents. *Archives of Disease in Childhood* 80, 406–409.

Carney, O., McIntosh, J. & Worth, A. (1996) The use of the nominal group technique in research with community nurses. *Journal of Advanced Nursing* 23(5), 1024–1029.

Catling, H. & Rodgers, P. (1971) Forecasting the textile scene: an aid to the planning of a research programme. *R&D Management* 1(3), 141–146.

Caulfield, T. & Chapman, A. (2005) Human dignity as a criterion for science policy. *Public Library of Science Medicine* 2(8), e244.

Cavalli-Sforza, V. & Ortolano, L. (1984) Delphi forecasts of land-use – transportation interactions. *Journal of Transportation Engineering* 110(3), 324–339.

Caves, R. (1988) Consultative methods for extracting expert knowledge about clinical competence. In: *Professional Competence and Quality Assurance in the Caring Professions* (Ed., R. Ellis). Chapman Hall, London, pp. 199–299.

Cawley, N. & Webber, J. (1995) Research priorities in palliative care. *International Journal of Palliative Nursing* 1(2), 101–113.

Chaffin, V.W. & Talley, W.K. (1980) Individual stability in Delphi studies. *Technological Forecasting and Social Change* 16, 67–73.

Chan, S. (1982) Expert judgment under uncertainty: some evidence and suggestions. *Social Science Quarterly* 63, 428–444.

Chang, E. & Daly, J. (1998) Priority areas for clinical research in palliative care nursing. *International Journal of Nursing Practice* 4(4), 247–253.

Chang, E., Ho, C.K., Yuen, A.C. & Hatcher, D. (2003) A study of clinical nursing research priorities in aged care: a Hong Kong perspective. *Contemporary Nurse* 15(3), 188–198.

Chien, I., Cook, S.W. & Harding, J. (1984) The field of American research. *American Psychologist* 3, 43–50.

Churchman, C.W. (1948) *Theory of Experimental Inference.* Macmillan Company, New York.

Churchman, C.W. (1973) *The Design of Inquiring Systems.* Basic Books, New York.

Clark, A. & Friedman, M.J. (1982) The relative importance of treatment outcomes. *Evaluation Review* 6, 79–93.

Clayton, M.J. (1997) Delphi: a technique to harness expert opinion for critical decision-making tasks in education. *Educational Psychology* 17(4), 373–386.

Cleary, K.K. (2001) Using the Delphi process to reach consensus. *Cardiopulmonary Physical Therapy Journal* 1, 20–23.

Cochran, S.W. (1983) The Delphi method: formulating and refining group judgments. *Journal of Human Sciences* 2(2), 111–117.

Cohen, M.Z., Harle, M. & Woll, A.M. (2004) Delphi survey of nursing research priorities. *Oncology Nursing Forum* 31, 1011–1018.

Cooney, C.F., Stebbings, S.N., Roxburgh, M., Mayo, J., Keen, N., Evans, E. & Meehan, T.C. (1995) Integrating nursing research and practice: Part II – a Delphi study of nursing practice priorities for research-based solutions. *Nursing Praxis in New Zealand* 10, 22–27.

Cornick, P. (2006) Nitric oxide education survey – use of a Delphi survey to produce guidelines for training neonatal nurses to work with inhaled nitric oxide. *Journal of Neonatal Nursing* 12(2), 62–68.

Couper, M.R. (1984) The Delphi technique: characteristics and sequence model. *ANS Advances in Nursing Science* 7(1), 72–77.

Creswell, J. (1994) *Research Design: Qualitative and Quantitative Approaches.* Sage Publications, Thousand Oaks, California.

Creswell, J. (2003) *Research Design. Qualitative, Quantitative and Mixed Methods Approaches.* Sage, Thousand Oaks, California.

Crisp, J., Pelletier, D., Duffield, C., Adams, A. & Nagy, S. (1997) The Delphi method? *Nursing Research* 46(2), 116–118.

Crisp, J., Pelletier, D., Duffield, C., Nagy, S. & Adams, A. (1999) Its all in a name: when is a Delphi study' not a Delphi study? *Australian Journal of Advanced Nursing* 16(3), 32–37.

Critcher, C. & Gladstone, B. (1998) Utilizing the Delphi technique in policy discussion: a case study of a privatized utility in Britain. *Public Administration* 76(3), 431–449.

Cronin, S.N. & Owsley, V.B. (1993) Identifying nursing research priorities in an acute care hospital. *Journal of Nursing Administration* 23(11), 58–62.

Cross, V. (1999) The same but different: a Delphi study of clinicians' and academics' perceptions of physiotherapy undergraduates. *Physiotherapy* 85(1), 28–39.

Crotty, M. (1998) *The Foundations of Social Research, Meaning and Perspective in the Research Process.* Delphi (Document No P3704), Sage, Thousand Oaks, California.

Cuhls, K., Blind, K. & Grupp, H. (2002) *Innovations for our Future. Delphi '98: New Foresight on Science and Technology.* Physica, Springer, Heidelberg, New York.

Custer, R.L., Scarcella, J.A. & Stewart, B.R. (1999) The modified Delphi technique – a rotational modification. *Journal of Vocational and Technical Education* 15(2), 50–58.

Cyphert, F.R. & Gant, W.L. (1970) The Delphi technique. *Journal of Teacher Education* 21(3), 422.

Cyphert, F.R. & Gant, W.L. (1971) The Delphi technique: a case study. *Phi Delta Kappan* 52, 272–273.

Czinkota, M.R. & Ronkainen, I.A. (1997) International business and trade in the next decade: report from a Delphi study. *Journal of International Business* 28(4), 827–844.

Dahl, A.W. (1974) *Delphic and Interactive Committee Processes in a Comprehensive Health Planning Advisory Council: A Comparative Case Study.* Unpublished PhD Thesis, Baltimore, MD; Johns Hopkins University School of Hygiene and Public health.

Dajani, J.S., Sincoff, M.Z. & Talley, W.K. (1979) Stability and agreement criteria for the termination of Delphi studies. *Technological Forecasting and Social Change* 13, 83–90.

Dalkey, N. & Helmer, O. (1962) *An Experimental Application of the Delphi Method to the Use of Experts.* Memorandum No RM-727/1-Abridged. The RAND Corporation, Santa Monica, California.

Dalkey, N. & Helmer, O. (1963) Delphi technique: characteristics and sequence model to the use of experts. *Management Science* 9(3), 458–467.

Dalkey, N.C. (1967) *Delphi.* Document No. P3704. The RAND Corporation, Santa Monica, California.

Dalkey, N.C. (1969a) *The Delphi Method: an Experimental Study of Group Opinion.* Document No RM-5888-PR. The RAND Corporation, Santa Monica, California.

Dalkey, N.C. (1969b) An experimental study of group opinion: the Delphi method. *Futures* 1(5), 408–426.

Dalkey, N.C. (1969c) Analysis from a group opinion. *Futures* 1(6), 541–551.

Dalkey, N.C. (1971) *Comparison of Group Judgement Techniques with Short-Range Predictions and Almanac Questions.* Document No R-678. The RAND Corporation, New York.

Dalkey, N.C. (1975) Toward a theory of group estimation. In: *The Delphi Method: Techniques and Applications* (Eds H.L. Linstone & M. Turoff). Addison-Wesley, Reading, Massachusetts, pp. 236–261.

Dalkey, N.C., Brown, B. & Cochran, S. (1969) *The Delphi Method III: Use of Self-Ratings to Improve Group Estimates.* Document No RM-6115-PR. The RAND Corporation, Santa Monica, California.

Dalkey, N.C., Brown, B. & Cochran, S. (1970) *The Delphi Method IV: Effects of Percentile Feedback and Feed-in of Relevant Facts.* Document No RM-6118-PR. The RAND Corporation, Santa Monica, California.

Daly, J., Chang, E.M. & Bell, P.F. (1996) Clinical nursing research priorities in Australian critical care: a pilot. *Journal of Advanced Nursing* 23(1), 145–151.

Daniels, L. & Ascough, A. (1999) Developing a strategy for cancer nursing research: identifying priorities. *European Journal of Oncology Nursing* 3(3), 161–169.

Daniels, L. & Howlett, C. (2001) The way forward: identifying palliative nursing research priorities within a hospice. *International Journal of Palliative Nursing* 7(9), 442–448.

Davidson, P., Merritt-Gray, M., Buchanan, J. & Noel, J. (1997) Voices from practice: mental health nurses identify research priorities. *Archives of Psychiatric Nursing* XI(6), 340–345.

Day, J. & Bobeva, M. (2004) Seeking the truth: The use of Delphi studies for IS research. In: *Reflection on the Past, Making Sense of Today and Predicting the Future of Information Systems* (Eds, K. Grant, D.A. Edgar & M. Jordan), 9th Annual UKAIS Conference Proceedings Annual Conference, 5–7 May 2004, Glasgow Caledonian University, Glasgow.

Day, J. & Bobeva, M. (2005) A generic toolkit for the successful management of Delphi studies. *The Electronic Journal of Business Research Methodology* 3(2), 103–116.

De Meyrick, J. (2003) The Delphi method and health research. *Health Education* 103(1), 7–16.

De Villiers, M.R., de Villiers, P.J.T. & Kent, A.P. (2005) The Delphi technique in health sciences education research. *Medical Teacher* 27(7), 639–643.

Delbecq, A.L., Van de Ven, A. & Gustafson, D. (1975) *Group Techniques for Program Planning: A Guide to Normal Group and Delphi Processes.* Scott, Foreman and Company, Glenview, Illinois.

Demi, A.S., Meredith, C.E. & Gray, M. (1996) Research priorities for urologic nursing: a Delphi study. *Urologic Nursing* 16(1), 3–7.

Dennis, K.E., Howes, D.G. & Zelauskas, B. (1989) Identifying nursing research priorities: a first step in program development. *Applied Nursing Research* 2(3), 108–113.

Denscombe, M. (2003) *The Good Research Guide: For Small-Scale Social Research Projects* (2nd Edn). Open University Press, Maidenhead.

Department of Health (1999) *National Service Framework for Mental Health.* Her Majesty's Stationery Office, London.

Department of Health and Children (1994) *Shaping a Healthier Future*. Department of Health and Children, Dublin.

Department of Health and Children (1998) *The Commission on Nursing*. Department of Health and Children, Dublin.

Derian, J.-C. & Morize, F. (1973) Delphi in the assessment of research and development projects. *Futures* 5(5), 469–483.

DeVon, H.A., Block, M.E., Moyle-Wright, P., Ernst, D.M., Hayden, S.J., Lazzara, D.J. Savoy, S.M. & Kostas-Polston, E. (2007) A psychometric toolbox for testing validity and reliability. *Journal of Nursing Scholarship* 39(2), 155–164.

Dewolfe, J.A., Laschinger, S. & Perkin, C. (2010) Preceptors' perspectives on recruitment, support, and retention of preceptors. *Journal of Nursing Education* 4, 1–9.

Diamond, B. (1998) Crisis in midwifery staffing: the legal aspects. *British Journal of Midwifery* 6, 755–757.

Dillman, D.A. (1978) *Mail and Telephone Surveys: The Total Design Method*. Wiley, New York.

Donabedian A. (1988) *The Quality of Care: How Can it Be Assessed? Journal of the American Medical Association* 260, 743–1748. In: A proposed conceptual framework for performance assessment in primary health care: a tool for policy and practice. Sibthorpe, B. (2004) *Canberra: Australian Primary Health Care Research Institute*. Available online: http://www.anu.edu.au/aphcri/Publications/conceptual_framework.pdf [accessed 10 July 2009].

Donohoe, H.M. & Needham, R.D. (2008) Moving best practice forward: Delphi characteristics, advantages, potential problems and solutions. *International Journal of Tourism Research* 11, 415–437.

Doughty, E. (2009) Investigating adaptive grieving styles: a Delphi study. *Death Studies* 33(5), 462–480.

Dransfeld, H., Pemberton, J. & Jacobs, G. (2000) Quantifying weighted expert opinion: the future of interactive television and retailing. *Technology Forecasting and Social Change* 63(1), 81–90.

Drennan, J., Meehan, T., Kemple, M., Johnson, M., Treacy, M. & Butler, M. (2007) Nursing research priorities for Ireland. *Nursing Scholarship* 39(4), 298–305.

Duffield, C. (1993) The Delphi technique: a comparison of results obtained using two expert panels. *International Journal of Nursing Studies* 30(3), 227–237.

Duncan, E.A.S., Nicol, M.M. & Age, A. (2004) Factors that constitute a good cognitive behavioural treatment manual: a Delphi study. *Behavioural and Cognitive Psychotherapy* 32(2), 199–213.

Dwyer, M. (1999) A Delphi study of research priorities and identified areas for collaborative research in health sector library and information services UK. *Health Libraries Review* 16, 174–191.

Eckman, C.A. (1983) *Development of an Instrument to Evaluate Intercollegiate Athletic Coaches: A Modified Delphi Study*. Unpublished doctoral dissertation, West Virginia University, Morgantown.

Edwards, L.H. (2002) Research priorities in school nursing: a Delphi process. *Journal of School Health* 72(5), 173–177.

Edwards, P., Roberts, I., Clarke, M., DiGuiseppi, C., Pratap, S., Wentz, R. & Kwan, I. (2002) Increasing response rates to postal questionnaires: systematic review. *British Medical Journal* 324, 1183–1185.

Efstathiou, N., Ameen, J. & Coll, A.M. (2007) Healthcare providers' priorities for cancer care: a Delphi study in Greece. *European Journal of Oncology Nursing* 11(2), 141–150.

Efstathiou, N., Ameen, J. & Coll, A.-M. (2008) A Delphi study to identify healthcare users' priorities for cancer care in Greece. *European Journal of Oncology Nursing* 12, 362–371.

Eggers, R.M. & Jones, C.M. (1998) Practical considerations for conducting Delphi studies: the oracle enters a new age. *Educational Research Quarterly* 21(3), 53–66.

Endacott, R. (1998) Needs of the critically ill child: a review of the literature and report of a modified Delphi study. *Intensive Critical Care Nursing* 14(2), 66–73.

Engles, T. & Kennedy, P.H. (2007) Enhancing a Delphi study on family-focused prevention. *Technological Forecasting and Social Change* 74(4), 433–451.

Errfmeyer, R.C., Erffmeyer, E.S. & Lane, I.M. (1986) The Delphi technique: an empirical evaluation of the optimum number of rounds. *Group and Organisational Studies* 11(1–2), 120–128.

Evans, C. (1997) The use of consensus methods and expert panels in pharmacoeconomic studies. Practical applications and methodological shortcomings. *Pharmacoeconomics* 12(2 Pt.1), 121–129.

Everett, A. (1993) Piercing the veil of the future: a review of the Delphi method of research. *Professional Nurse* 9, 181–185.

Farrell, P. & Scherer, K. (1983) The Delphi technique as a method for selecting criteria to evaluate nursing care. *Nursing Papers (Canada)* 15(1), 51–60.

Fawcett-Henesy, A. (1999) *Presentation Given at an All-Ireland Seminar on Public Health Nursing.* Canal Court Hotel, Newry, Co Down, Northern Ireland.

Fenwick, J., Butt, J., Downie, J., Monterosso, L. & Wood, J. (2006) Priorities for midwifery research in Perth, Western Australia: a Delphi study. *International Journal of Nursing Practice* 12(2), 78–93.

Ferguson, F., Brownlee, M. & Webster, V. (2008) A Delphi study investigating consensus among expert physiotherapists in relation to the management of low back pain. *Musculoskeletal Care* 6(4), 197–210.

Field, A. (2005) *Discovering Statistics Using SPSS.* Sage Publications, London.

Fink, A., Kosecoff, J., Cassinm M. & Brook, R. H. (1984) Consensus methods: characteristics and guidelines for use. *American Journal of Public Health* 74, 979–983.

Fisher, R.G. (1978) The Delphi method: a description, review and criticism. *Journal of Academic Librarianship* 4, 64–70.

Fitzpatrick, E., Sullivan, J., Smith, A., Mucowski, D., Hoffman, E., Dunn, P., Trice, M. & Grosso, L. (1991) Clinical nursing research priorities: a Delphi study. *Clinical Nurse Specialist* 5(2), 94–99.

Fitzsimmons J.A. & Fitzsimmons, M.J. (2001) *Service Management: Operations, Strategy and Information Technology* (4th Edn). McGraw-Hill, Boston.

Fochtman, D. & Hinds, P. (2000) Identifying nursing research priorities in a pediatric clinical trials cooperative group: the pediatric oncology group experience. *Journal of Pediatric Oncology Nursing* 17(2), 83–87.

Fontenrose, J. (1978) *The Delphic Oracle, Its Responses and Operations with a Catalouge of Responses.* University of California Press, Berkeley.

Forte, P.S., Ritz, L.J. & Balestracci, J.M.S. (1997) Identifying nursing research priorities in a newly merged healthcare system. *Journal of Nursing Administration* 27, 51–55.

Francis, A. (1977) An experimental analysis of a Delphi technique: the effect of majority and high confidence-low confidence expert opinion on group consensus. *Dissertation Abstracts International* 38(02), 566.

Francomb, H. (1997) Do we need HCA's in the maternity services? *British Journal of Midwifery* 5, 672–679.

Franklin, K.K. & Hart, J.K. (2007) Idea generation and exploration: benefits and limitations of the policy Delphi research method. *Innovative Higher Education* 31(4), 237–246.

French, P., Ho, Y. & Lee, L. (2002) A Delphi survey of evidence-based nursing priorities in Hong Kong. *Journal of Nursing Management* 10, 265–273.

Garrod, B. & Fyall, A. (2005) Revisiting Delphi: the Delphi technique research. In: *Tourism Research Methods: Integrating Theory and Practice* (Eds, B.W. Richiem, P. Burns & C. Palmer). CAB International, Wallingford, pp. 85–98.

Geist, M. (2009) Using the Delphi method to engage stakeholders: a comparison of two studies. *Evaluation and Program Planning* 23(2), 147–154.

Gerein, N., Green, A. & Pearson, S. (2006) The implications of shortages of health professionals for maternal health in sub-Saharan Africa. *Reproductive Health Matters* 14(27), 40–50.

Gibbs, A. (1997) Focus Groups. *Social Research Update.* Issue 19 Available online: http://sru.soc.surrey.ac.uk/SRU19.html [accessed 28 July 2009]

Gibson, J.M.E. (1998) Using the Delphi to identify the content and context of nurses continuing professional development needs. *Journal of Clinical Nursing* 7, 451–459.

Gibson, (2001) *Cooperative Extension Program Planning in Wisconsin.* Program Development and Evaluation. University of Wisconsin-Extension Cooperative Extension Madison, Wisconsin.

Goodman, C. (1986) *A Delphi Survey of Clinical Nursing Research Priorities Within a Regional Health Authority.* Unpublished MSc Thesis, University of London, London.

Goodman, C.M. (1987) The Delphi technique: a critique. *Journal of Advanced Nursing* 12, 729–734.

Gordon, T.J. (1992) The methods in futures research. *Annals of the American Academy of Political and Social Science* 522, 25–35.

Gordon, T.J. (1994) *The Delphi Method.* AC/UNU Millennium Project, Futures Research Methodology. Available online: http://www.gerenciamento. ufba.br/Downloads/delphi%20(1).pdf [accessed 16 August 2010].

Gordon, T.J. & Helmer, O. (1964) *Report on a Long-Range Forecasting Study.* Document No P-2982, The RAND Corporation, Santa Monica, California.

Graduate Medical Education National Advisory Committee (1980) *The Report of the Graduate Medical Educational National Advisory Committee.* Vols I-VII, USDHHS Pub Nos (HRA) 81-651 to 81-657. Government Printing Office, Washington, DC.

Graham, B., Regehr, G. & Wright, J.G. (2003) Delphi as a method to establish consensus for diagnostic criteria. *Journal of Clinical Epidemiology* 56, 1150–1156.

Greatorex, J. & Dexter, T. (2000) An accessible analytical approach for investigating what happens between the rounds of a Delphi study. *Journal of Advanced Nursing* 32, 1016–1024.

Green, B., Jones, M., Hughes, D. & Williams, A. (1999) Applying the Delphi technique in a study of GPs information requirement. *Health and Social Care in the Community* 7(3), 198–205.

Green, H., Hunter, C. & Moore, B. (1990) Application of the Delphi technique in tourism. *Annals of Tourism Research* 17(2), 270–279.

Green, J.P. (1982) *The Content of a College-Level Outdoor Leadership Course.* Paper presented at the Conference of the Northwest District Association for the American Alliance for Health, Physical Education, Recreation, and Dance, Spokane, WA, United States.

Griffin-Sobel, J.P. & Suozzo, S. (2002) Nursing research priorities for the care of the clinet with a gastrointestinal disorder: a Delphi survey. *Gastroenterology Nursing* 25(5), 188–191.

Grimes, R. & Moseley, S.K. (1976) An approach to an index of hospital performance. *Health Services Research* (Fall) 288–301.

Grundy, M. & Ghazi, F. (2009) Research priorities in haemato-oncology nursing: results of a literature review and a Delphi study. *European Journal of Oncology Nursing* 13(4), 235–249.

Guba, E. & Lincoln, Y. (1998) Competing paradigms in qualitative research. In: *The Landscape of Qualitative Research: Theories and Issues* (Eds, N. Denzin & Y. Lincoln). Sage, Thousand Oaks, California, pp. 195–220.

Guba, E.G. & Lincoln, Y.A. (1989) *Fourth Generation Evaluation.* Sage, Newbury Park, California.

Gupta, U.G. & Clarke, R.E. (1996) Theory and applications of the Delphi technique: a bibliography (1975–1994). *Technological Forecasting and Social Change* 53, 185–211.

Gutierrez, O. (1989) Experimental techniques for information requirements analysis. *Information and Management* 16, 31–34.

Hanafin, S. (2004) *Review of Literature on the Delphi Technique.* The National Children's Office, Dublin, Ireland.

Hanafin, S. (2005) *The Delphi Technique: A Methodology to Support the Development of a Nationals Set of Child Well-Being Indicators.* The National Children's Office, Dublin, Ireland.

Hardy, D.J., O'Brien, A.P., Gaskin, C.J., O'Brien, A.J., Morrison-Ngatai, E., Skews, G., Ryan, T. & McNulty, N. (2004) Practical application of the Delphi technique in bicultural mental health nursing study in New Zealand. *Journal of Advanced Nursing* 46(1), 95–109.

Hasson, F., Keeney, S. & McKenna, H. (2000) Research guidelines for the Delphi survey technique. *Journal of Advanced Nursing* 32(4), 1008–1015.

Hatton, J.M. & Nunnelee, J.D. (1995) Research priorities in vascular nursing. *Journal of Vascular Nursing* 13, 1–7.

Hauck, Y., Kelly, R.G. & Fenwick, J. (2007) Research priorities for parenting and child health: a Delphi study. *Journal of Advanced Nursing* 59(2), 129–139.

Heffline, M., Clark, M.L., Hooper, V.D, Mamaril, M., Miller, K.M., Norris, S., Poole, E.L., Summers, S. & Younger, S. (1994) Research priorities for all phases of postanesthesia nursing: a survey by ASPAN. *Journal of Postanesthesia Nursing* 9(4), 204–213.

Helmer, O. (1963) *The Systematic Use of Expert Judgment in Operations Research.* Document No P2795, The RAND Corporation, Santa Monica, California.

Helmer, O. (1964) *Convergence of Expert Consensus through Feedback.* The RAND Corporation, Santa Monica, California.

Helmer, O. (1967) *Systematic Use of Expert Opinions* (Document Number P-3721). The RAND Corporation, Santa Monica, California.

Helmer, O. (1975) Foreword. In: *The Delphi Method: Techniques and Applications* (Eds, H.A. Linstone & M. Turoff). Addison-Wesley, Massachusetts.

Helmer, O. (1977) Problems in futures research: Delphi and casual cross-impact analysis. *Futures* 9, 17–31.

Helmer, O. & Quade, E.S. (1963) *An Approach to the Study of a Developing Economy by Operational Gaming.* Document No P2718 The RAND Corporation, Santa Monica California.

Helmer, O. & Rescher, N. (1959) On epistemology of inexact sciences. *Management Science* 6(10), 25–52.

Henry, B., Moody, L.E., Pendergast, J.F., O'Donnell, J., Hutchinson, S.A. & Scully, G. (1987) Delineation of nursing administration research priorities. *Nursing Research* 36(5), 309–314.

Henschke, N., Maher, C., Refshauge, K., Das, A. & McAuley, J.H. (2007) Low back pain research priorities: a survey of primary care practitioners. *BMC Family Practice* 8, 40. Available online: http://www.biomedcentral.com/1471-2296/8/40 [accessed 26 February 2010].

Hermann, R., Mattke, S., Somekh, S., Silfverhielm, H., Goldner, E., Glover, G., Pirkis, J., Maniz, J. & Chan, J. (2006) Quality indicators for international benchmarking of mental health care. *International Journal for Quality in Health Care* 18(Suppl 1), 31–38.

Hicks, C. (1999) *Research Methods for Clinical Therapists: Applied Project Design and Analysis.* Churchill Livingstone, Edinburgh.

Hill, K.Q. & Fowles, J. (1975) The methodological worth of the Delphi forecasting technique. *Technological Forecasting and Social Change* 7, 179–192.

Hinds, P.S., Norville, R., Anthony, L.K., Briscoe, B.W., Gattuso, J.S., Quargnenti, A., Riggins, M.S., Walters, L.A., Wentz, L.J., Scarbrough, K.E. & Fairdough, D. (1990) Establishing pediatric cancer nursing research priorities: a Delphi study. *Journal of Pediatric Oncology Nursing* 7(3), 101–108.

Hinds, P.S., Quargnenti, A., Olson, M.S., Gross, J., Puckett, P., Randall, E., Gattuso, J.S. & Wiedenhoffer, D. (1994) The 1992 APON Delphi study to establish research priorities for pediatric oncology nursing. Association of Pediatric Oncology Nurses. *Journal of Pediatric Oncology Nursing* 11(1), 20–27.

Hitch, P.J. & Murgatroyd, J.D. (1983) Professional communications in cancer care: a Delphi survey of hospital nurses. *Journal of Advanced Nursing* 8, 413–422.

Holey, E.A., Feeley, J.L., Dixon, J. & Whittaker, V.J. (2007) An exploration in the use of simple statistics to measure consensus and stability in Delphi studies. *BMC Medical Research Methodology* 7, 52. Available online: http://www.ncbi.nlm.nih.gov/pmc/articles/PMC2216026/ [accessed 18 February 2010].

Holloway, I. & Wheeler, S. (1996) *Qualitative Research for Nurses*. Blackwell Science, Oxford.

Hope, G. (1977) *An Empirical Investigation to Identify Continuing Education Needs for Nurses in a National Health Agency*. Unpublished doctoral dissertation, Catholic University of America, United States.

Hsu, C.C. & Sandford, B.A. (2007) The Delphi technique: making sense of consensus. *Practical Assessment, Research and Evaluation* 12(10), 1–8.

Huang, H.-C., Lin, W.-C. & Lin, J.-D. (2008) Development of a fall-risk checklist using the Delphi technique. *Journal of Clinical Nursing* 17(17), 2275–2283.

Huckfeldt, V.E. & Judd, R.C. (1974) Issues in large scale Delphi studies. *Technological Forecasting and Social Change* 6, 75–88.

Hung, H.-L., Altschuld, J.W. & Lee, F.-Y. (2008) Methodological and conceptual issues confronting a cross-country Delphi study of educational program evaluation. *Evaluation and Program Planning* 21(2), 191–198.

Irish Nurses Organisation (1999a) *Official Notice to Members*. Irish Nurses Organisation, Dublin.

Irish Nurses Organisation (1999b) *Executive Council Policy Statement*. Irish Nurses Organisation, Dublin.

Ishikawa, A., Amagasa, M., Shiga, T., Tomizawa, G., Tatsuta, R. & Mieno, H. (1993) The max-min Delphi method and fuzzy Delphi method via fuzzy integration. *Fuzzy Sets and Systems* 55(3), 241–253.

Jacobs, J.M. (1996) *Essential Assessment Criteria for Physical Education Teacher Education Programs: A Delphi Study*. Unpublished doctoral dissertation, West Virginia University, Morgantown.

Jairath, N. & Weinstein, J. (1994) The Delphi Methodology (part one): a useful administrative approach. *Canadian Journal of Nursing Administration* 7(3), 29–40.

Jeffery, G., Hache, G. & Lehr, R. (1995) A group based Delphi application: defining rural career counselling needs. *Measurement and Evaluation in Counselling and Development* 28, 45–60.

Jenkins, D. & Smith, T. (1994) Applying Delphi methodology in family therapy research. *Contemporary Family Therapy* 16(5), 411–430.

Jillson, I. (1975a) Developing guidelines for the Delphi method. *Technological Forecasting and Social Change* 7(2), 221–222.

Jillson, I.A. (1975b) The national drug-abuse policy Delphi. In: *The Delphi Method, Techniques and applications* (Eds, H.A. Linstone & M. Turoff). Addison-Wesley, Reading, Massachusetts, pp. 124–159.

Jolson, M.A. & Rossow, G.L. (1971) The Delphi Process in marketing decision making. *Journal of Marketing Research* 8, 443–448.

Jones, F., Rice, V., Brown, P., Newman B., Malcolm P., Gilmour J., *et al.* (1989) *Clinical Nursing Research Priorities of Community Nurses in Western Sydney*. New South Wales Nurses Research Interest Group Conference Proceedings, Sydney, Australia.

Jones, H. & Twiss, B.C. (1978) *Forecasting Technology for Planning Decisions*. Petrocelli Books, New York.

Jones, J. & Hunter, D. (1995) Consensus methods for medical and health services research. *British Medical Journal* 311, 376–380.

Jones, J.M.G., Sanderson, C.F.B. & Black, N.A. (1992) What will happen to the quality of care with fewer junior doctors? A Delphi study of consultant physicians' views. *Journal of the Royal College of Physicians London* 26, 36–40.

Jorm, A.F., Minas, H., Langlands, R.L. & Kelly, C.M. (2008) First aid guidelines for psychosis in Asian countries: a Delphi consensus study. *International Journal of Mental Health Systems* 2(1), 2.

Judd, R.C. (1972) Use of Delphi methods in higher education. *Technological Forecasting and Social Change* 4(2), 173–186.

Jung-Erceg, P., Pandza, K., Armbruster, H. & Dreher, C. (2007) Absorptive capacity in European manufacturing: a Delphi study. *Industrial Management and Data Systems* 107(1), 37–51.

Jurkovich, G., Rivara, F., Johansen, J. & Maier, R. (2004) Centers for Disease Control and Prevention injury research agenda: identification of acute care research topics of interest to the Centers for Disease Control and Prevention – National Center for Injury Prevention and Control. *Journal of Trauma* 56, 1166–1170.

Kahneman, D., Slovic, P. & Tversky, A. (1982) *Judgment under Uncertainty: Heuristics and Biases.* Cambridge University Press, Cambridge.

Kaplan, A., Skogstad, A.L. & Girshick, M. (1949) *The Prediction of Social Technological Events.* Document No P93, The RAND Corporation, Santa Monica, California.

Kaplan, L.M. (1971) *The Use of the Delphi Method in Organizational Communication: A Case Study.* Unpublished master's thesis, The Ohio State University, Columbus.

Kastein, M.R., Jacobs, M., Van Der Hell, R.H., Luttik, K. & Touw-Otten, F.W.M.M. (1993) Delphi, the issue of reliability: a qualitative Delphi study in primary health care in the Netherlands. *Technological Forecasting and Social Change* 44, 315–323.

Kaynak, E. & Marandu, E.E. (2006) Tourism market potential analysis in Botswana: a Delphi study. *Journal of Travel Research* 45, 227–237.

Keeney, S. (2009) *The Delphi Technique in: The Research Process in Nursing* (Eds, K. Gerrish & A. Lacey) (6th Edn). Blackwell Publishing, London.

Kelly, K.P. & Porock, D. (2005) A survey of pediatric oncology nurses' perceptions of parent educational needs. *Journal of Pediatric Oncology Nursing* 22(1), 58–66.

Keeney, S., Hasson, F. & McKenna, H.P. (2001) A critical review of the Delphi technique as a research methodology for nursing. *International Journal of Nursing Studies* 38, 195–200.

Keeney, S., Hasson, F. & McKenna, H.P. (2006) Consulting the oracle: ten lessons from using the Delphi technique in nursing research. *Journal of Advanced Nursing* 53(2), 205–212.

Kennedy, P.H. (2004) Enhancing Delphi research: methods and results. *Journal of Advanced Nursing* 45(5), 504–511.

Kilroy, D. & Driscoll, P. (2006) Determination of required anatomical knowledge for clinical practice in emergency medicine: national curriculum planning using a modified Delphi technique. *Journal of Emergency Medicine* 23, 693–696.

Kim, M.J., Oh, E., Kim, C., Yoo, J. & Ko, I. (2002) Priorities for nursing research in Korea. *Journal of Nursing Scholarship* 34, 307–312.

Kim, M., Eui-Geum, O., Cho-Ja, K., Ji-Soo, Y. & Il-Sun, K. (2004) Priorities for nursing research in Korea. *Journal of Nursing Scholarship* 34(4), 307–312.

Kirkwood, M., Wales, A. & Wilson, A. (2003) A Delphi study to determine nursing research priorities in the North Glasgow University Hospitals NHS Trust and the corresponding evidence base. *Health Information and Libraries Journal* 20(1), 53–80.

Klessig, J.M., Wolfsthal, S.D., Levine, M.A., Sfickley, W., Bing-You, R.G., Lansdale, T.F. & Battinelli, D.L. (2000) A pilot survey study to define quality in residency education. *Academic Medicine* 75, 71–73.

Klimenko, E. & Julliard, K. (2007) Communication between CAM and mainstream medicine: Delphi panel perspectives. *Complementary Therapies in Clinical Practice* 13(1), 46–52.

Koopman, W., Avolio, J., Wong, C., Davies, K., Dennis, K., Fisher, P. & Morgan, S. (1995) Identifying nursing research priorities: general and neuroscience specific at an acute care hospital. *Axone* 17(1), 9–15.

Krefting, L. (1991) Rigour in qualitative research: the assessment of trustworthiness. *American Journal of Occupational Therapy* 45(3), 214–222.

Kuusi, O. (1999) *Expertise in the Future Use of Generic Technologies: Epistemic and Methodological Considerations Concerning Delphi Studies.* Government Institute for Economical Research VATT, Helsinki.

Landeta, J. (2006) Current validity of the Delphi method in social sciences. *Technological Forecasting and Social Change* 73, 467–482.

Lang, T. (1994) *An Overview of Four Futures Methodologies.* Available online: http://www.futures.hawaii.edu/j7/LANG.html [accessed 18 February 2010].

Lathlean, J. (2005) Qualitative analysis. In: *The Research Process in Nursing* (Eds, K. Gerrish & A. Lacey) (5th Edn). Blackwell Publishing, Oxford, pp. 417–433.

Leang, S. (2008) The impact of the HIV epidemic on health services in Cambodia: a Delphi study. *Asia Pacific Journal of Public Health* 20(Suppl), 141–147.

Lemmer, B. (1998) Successive surveys of an expert panel: research in decision making with health visitors. *Journal of Advanced Nursing* 27, 538–545.

Lewandowski, L.A. & Kositsky, A.M. (1983) Research priorities for critical care nursing. *Heart and Lung* 12(1), 34–44.

Lewis, S.L., Cooper, C.L., Cooper, K.G., Bonner, P.N., Parker, K. & Frauman, A. (1999) Research priorities for nephrology nursing: American Nephrology Nurses' Association's Delphi Study. *American Nephrology Nurses' Association Journal* 26(2), 215–225.

Lincoln, Y.S. & Guba, E.G. (1985) *Naturalistic Inquiry.* Sage Publications Inc: New Bury Park, London.

Lindeman, C. (1974) *Delphi Survey of Clinical Nursing Research Priorities.* Western Interstate Commission for Higher Education, Boulder, California.

Lindeman, C. (1975) Delphi survey of priorities in clinical nursing research. *Nursing Research* 24, 434–441.

Lindquist, R., Banasik, J., Barnsteiner, J., Beecroft, P.C., Prevost, S., Riegel, B., Sechrist, K., Strzeleecki, C. & Titler, M. (1993) Determining AACN's research priorities for the 90s. *American Journal of Critical Care* 2(2), 110–117.

Linstone, H.A. (1975) Eight basic pitfalls: a checklist. In: *The Delphi Method: Techniques and Applications* (Eds, H.D. Linstone & M. Turoff). Addison-Wesley, Reading, Massachusetts, pp. 573–586.

Linstone, H.A. (1978) The Delphi technique. In: *Handbook of Futures Research* (Ed., J. Fowlers). Greenwood Press, Westport, pp. 273–300.

Linstone, H.A. (1999) *Decision Making for Technology Executives: Using Multiple Perspectives to Improve Performance.* Artech House, Boston, Massachusetts.

Linstone, H.A. & Turoff, M. (1975) *The Delphi Method: Techniques and Applications.* Addison-Wesley, Reading, Massachusetts.

Longhurst, R. (1971) *An Economic Evaluation of Human Resources Program with Respect to Pregnancy Outcome and Intellectual Development.* Cornell University, Ithaca, New York.

Loo, R. (2002) The Delphi method: a powerful tool for strategic management. *Policing an International Journal of Police Strategies and Management* 25(4), 762–769.

Lopez, V. (2003) Critical care nursing research priorities in Hong Kong. *Journal of Advanced Nursing* 43, 578–587.

Loughlin, K.G. & Moore, L.F. (1979) Using Delphi to achieve congruent objectives and activities in a pediatrics department, *Journal of Medical Education* 54(2), 101–106.

Love, C. (1997) A Delphi study examining standards for patient handling. *Nursing Standard* 11, 34–48.

Ludwing, B. (1997) Predicting the future: have you considered using the Delphi methodology? *Journal of Extension* 35(5) Available online: http://www.joe.org/joe/1997october/tt2.php [accessed 16 August 2010].

Lynch, P., Jackson, M. & Saint, S. (2001) Research Priorities Project, year 2000: establishing a direction for infection control and hospital epidemiology. *American Journal of Infection Control* 29, 73–78.

Lynn, M.R., Layman, E.L. & Englebardt, S.P. (1998) Nursing administration research priorities: a national Delphi study. *Journal of Nursing Administration* 28(5), 7–11.

Macilraith, N. (1992) Clinical nursing research priorities: a Delphi study. *Association of Perioperative Registered Nurses* 56(2), 348–350.

Mackellar, A., Ashcroft, D.M., Bell, D., Higman James, D. & Marriott, J. (2007) Identifying criteria for the assessment of pharmacy students' communication skills with patients. *American Journal of Pharachological Education* 71(3), 50.

Macmillan, M., Atkinson, F. & Prophit, P. (1989) *A Delphi Survey of Priorities for Nursing Research in Scotland.* Nursing Studies Research Unit, University of Edinburgh, UK.

Madigan, E.A. & Vanderboom C. (2005) Home health care nursing research priorities. *Applied Nursing Research* 18(4), 221–225.

Malcolm, C., Knighting, K., Forbat, L. & Kearney, N. (2009) Prioritization of future research topics for children's hospice care by its key stakeholders: a Delphi study. *Palliative Medicine* 23(5), 398–405.

Malmsjö, A. (2006) A sketch of a methodology for designing supportive information systems. *Kybernetes* 35(6), 880–898.

Malone, D.C., Abarca, J., Hansten, P.D., Grizzle, A.J., Armstrong, E.P., Van Bergen, R.C., Duncan-Edgar, B.S., Solomon, S.L. & Lipton, R.B. (2005)

Identification of serious drug-drug interactions: results of the partnership to prevent drug-drug interactions. *American Journal of Geriatric Pharmacotherapy* 3(2), 65–76.

Mamaril, M., Ross, J., Poole, E.L., Brady, J.M. & Clifford, T. (2009) ASPAN's Delphi study on national research: priorities for perianesthesia nurses in the United States. *Journal of Perianesthesia Nursing* 24(1), 4–13.

Martino, J.P. (1993) *Technological Forecasting for Decision Making*. McGraw Hill, Dayton.

Mayaka, M. & King, B. (2002) A quality assessment of education and training for Kenya's tour operating sector. *Current Issue in Tourism* 5(2), 112–133.

McBride, A.J., Pates, R., Ramadan, R. & McGowan, C. (2003) Delphi survey of experts' opinions on strategies used by community pharmacists to reduce over-the-counter drug misuse. *Addiction* 98, 487–494.

Mcilfatrick, S.J. & Keeney, S. (2003) Identifying cancer nursing research priorities using the Delphi technique. *Journal of Advanced Nursing* 42(6), 629–636.

McIntire, S.A. & Miller, L.A. (2005) *Foundations of Psychological Testing*. Sage Publishing Company, London and New York.

McKee, M., Priest, P., Ginzler, M. & Black, N. (1991) How representative are members of expert panels. *Quality Assurance in Health Care* 3, 89–94.

McKenna, H., Hasson, F. & Smith, M. (2002) A Delphi survey of midwives and midwifery students to identify non-midwifery duties. *Midwifery* 18(4), 314–322.

McKenna, H.P. (1994a) The Delphi technique: a worthwhile approach for nursing? *Journal of Advanced Nursing* 19, 1221–1225.

McKenna, H.P. (1994b) The essential elements of a practitioners' nursing model: a survey of clinical psychiatric nurse managers. *Journal of Advanced Nursing* 19, 870–877.

McKenna, H.P. & Hasson, F. (2000) *A Review of Midwifery Skill Mix Within the Rotunda Hospital Dublin.* Unpublished report. Centre for Nursing Research, University of Ulster.

McKenna, H.P. & Hasson, F. (2001) A study of skills mix issues in midwifery: a multi-method approach. *Journal of Advanced Nursing* 37(1), 95–113.

McKenna, H.P. & Keeney, S. (2004) Leadership within community nursing in Ireland north and south: the perceptions of community nurses, GPs, policy makers and members of the public. *Journal of Nursing Management* 12, 69—76.

McKenna, H.P. & Keeney, S. (2008a) Commentary. *Journal of Clinical Nursing* 17, 2511–2520.

McKenna, H.P. & Keeney, S. (2008b) Delphi studies. In: *Nursing Research: Designs and Methods* (Eds, R. Watson, H.P. McKenna, S. Cowman & J. Keady). Churchill Livingstone, Edinburgh, pp. 251–260.

McKenna, H.P., Hasson, F. & Smith, M. (2001) A Delphi survey of midwives and midwifery students to identify non-midwifery duties. *Midwifery* 18, 314–322.

McKenna, H.P., Keeney, S. & Bradley, M. (2003) Generic and specialist nursing roles: views of community nurses, general practitioners, senior policy makers and members of the public. *Health and Social Care in the Community* 11(6), 537–545.

McKenna, H.P., Hasson, F. & Keeney, S.R. (2006) Surveys. In: *The Research Process in Nursing* (Eds, K. Gerrish & A. Lacey). Blackwell, Oxford, pp. 260–272.

McKeown, C. & Gibson, F. (2007) Determining the political influence of nurses who work in the field of hepatitis C: a Delphi survey. *Journal of Clinical Nursing* 16(7), 1210–1021.

McMurray, A.R. (1994) Three decision making aids – brainstorming, nominal group and the Delphi technique. *Journal of Nursing Staff Development* 10(2), 62–65.

McNally, J.A. (1974) *Toward Anticipating Possible Needs for Nursing Services That Might Emerge from Anticipated Social and Technological Developments: A Demonstration of the Use of the Delphi Method.* Unpublished doctoral dissertation, Columbia University, New York.

Mead, D. (1991) An evaluation tool for primary nursing. *Nursing Standard* 6(1), 37–39.

Mead, D. & Moseley, L. (2001) The use of Delphi as a research approach. *Nurse Researcher* 8(4), 23.

Meadows, A.B., Maine, L.L., Keyes, E.K., Pearson, K. & Finstuen, K. (2005) Pharmacy executive leadership issues and associated skills, knowledge and abilities. *Journal of American Pharmacists Association* 45(1), 55–62.

Miles, M.B. & Huberman, A.M. (1994) *Qualitative Data Analysis* (2nd Edn). Sage, Thousand Oaks, California.

Milholland, A.V., Wheeler, S.G. & Heieck, J.J. (1973) Medical assessment by a Delphi group opinion technique. *New England Journal of Medicine* 288, 1272–1275.

Miller, G. (2001) The development of indicators for sustainable tourism: results of a Delphi survey of tourism researchers. *Tourism Management* 22, 351–362.

Miller, L.E. (2006) *Determining What Could/Should Be: The Delphi Technique and Its Application.* Paper presented at the meeting of the 2006 annual meeting of the Mid-Western Educational Research Association, Columbus, Ohio.

Miller, W.L. & Crabtree, B.F. (1992) Primary care research: a multi-method typology and qualitative road map. In: *Doing Qualitative Research.* Vol. 3 (Eds, B.J. Crabtree & W.L. Miller). Sage, Newbury Park, California, pp. 3–30.

Misener, T.R., Alexander, J.W., Blaha, A.J., Clarke, P.N., Cover, C.M., Felton, G.M. Fuller, S.G., Herman, J., Rodes, M.M. & Sharp, H.F. (1997) National Delphi study to determine competencies for nursing leadership in public health. *Journal of Nursing Scholarship* 29(1), 47–51.

Mitchell, M.P. (1998) Nursing education planning: a Delphi study. *Journal of Nursing Education* 37(7), 305–307.

Mitchell, V.W. (1991) The Delphi technique: an exposition and application. *Technology Analysis and Strategic Management* 3(4), 333–358.

Mitroff A. & Turoff, M. (1975) Philosophical and methodological foundations of Delphi. Document No: P17–36. In: *The Delphi Method. Techniques and Applications* (Eds, H.A. Linstone & M. Turoff). Addison-Wesley, London, pp. 17–34.

Moeller, G.H. & Shafer, E.L. (1994) The Delphi technique a tool for long-range travel and tourism planning. In: *Travel, Tourism, and Hospitality Research. A Handbook for Managers and Researchers* (Eds, J.R.B. Richie & C.R. Goeldner). USDA Forest Service, Washington, DC, pp. 473–480.

Mohorjy, A.M. & Aburizaiza, O.S. (1997) Impact assessment of an improper effluent control system: a Delphi approach. *Environmental Impact Assessment Review* 17, 205–217.

Monterosso, L., Dadd, G., Ranson, K. & Toye, C. (2001) Priorities for paediatric cancer nursing research in Western Australia: a Delphi study. *Contemporary Nursing* 11(2–3), 142–152.

Monti, E.J. & Tingen, M.S. (1999) Multiple paradigms of nursing science. *Advanced in Nursing Science* 21(4), 64–80.

Moore, C.M. (1987) Delphi Technique and the mail questionnaire. In: *Group Techniques for Idea Building: Applied Social Research Methods* (Ed., C.M. Moore). Series 9, Sage Publications, Newbury Park, California, pp. 50–77.

Moreno-Casbas, T., Martin-Arribas, C., Orts-Cortes, I. & Comet-Cortes, P. (2001) Identification of priorities for nursing research in Spain: a Delphi study. *Journal of Advanced Nursing* 35, 857–863.

Morgan, B.C. (1982) Projecting physician requirements for child health care-1990. *Peadiatrics* 69, 150–156.

Morgan, D.L. (1998) Practical strategies for combining qualitative and quantitative methods: applications to health research. *Qualitative Health Research* 8(3), 362–376.

Morgan, P.J., Lam-McCullough, J., Herold-McIlroy, J. & Tarshis, J. (2007) Simulation performance checklist generation using the Delphi technique. *Canadian Journal of Anesthesia* 51(12), 992–997.

Moseley, L. & Mead, D. (2001) Considerations in using the Delphi approach design, questions and answers. *Nurse Researcher* 8(4), 24–37.

Mullen, P.M. (2000) *When Is Delphi Not Delphi?* Discussion Paper 37, Health Services Management Centre, University of Birmingham, Birmingham.

Mullen, P.M. (2003) Delphi: myths and reality. *Journal of Health Organization and Management* 17(1), 37–52.

Munier, F. & Ronde, P. (2001) The role of knowledge codification in the emergence of consensus under uncertainty: empirical analysis and policy implications. *Research Policy* 20, 1537–1551.

Murphy, M.K, Black, N.A., Lamping, D.L., McKee, C.M., Sanderson, C.F.B, Askham, J. & Marteau, T. (1998) Consensus development methods and their use in clinical guideline development. *Health Technology Assessment* 2(3), 1–88.

Murray, T.J. (1979) Delphi methodologies: a review and critique. *Urban Systems* 4(2), 153–158.

Murray, W.F. & Jarman, B.O. (1987) Predicting future trends in adult fitness using the Delphi approach. *Research Quarterly for Exercise and Sport* 58(2), 124–131.

Murry, J.W. & Hammons, J.O. (1995) Delphi: a versatile methodology for conducting qualitative research. *Review of Higher Education* 18, 423–436.

Mussallem, H.K. (1970) 2020: Nursing fifty years hence. In: *Nursing Education in a Changing Society* (Ed., M.Q. Innis). University of Toronto Press, Toronto, pp. 209–224.

Nappier, P., Stanfield, J., Simon, J.M., Bennett, S. & Cowan, C.F. (1990) Identifying clinical nursing research priorities. *Nursing Connections* 3(2), 45–50.

Nathens, A., Cook, C., Machiedo, G., Moore, E., Namias, N. & Nwariaku, F. (2006) Defining the research agenda for surgical infection: a consensus of experts using the Delphi approach. *Surgical Infections* 7, 101–110.

National Health Service Confederation and British Medical Association (2003) *New GMS Contract 2003 – Investing in General Practice.* NHS Confederation and BMA, London.

National Institute of Science and Technology Policy (1997) *The Sixth Technology Forecast Survey – Future Technology in Japan.* National Institute of Science and Technology Policy, Japan.

Naylor, C., Samele, C. & Wallcraft, J. (2008) Research priorities for 'patient-centered' mental health services: findings from a national consultation. *Mental Health Review Journal* 13(4), 33–43.

Needham, R.D. & de Loë, R. (1990) The policy Delphi: purpose, structure, and application. *The Canadian Geographer* 34(2), 133–142.

Newman, K., Maylor, U. & Chansarkar, B. (2001) The nurse retention, quality of care and patient satisfaction chain. *International Journal of Health Care Quality Assurance* 14(2), 57–68.

Nguyen, O., Higgs P. & Hellard, M. (2009) Limits to relying on expert information: the Delphi technique in a study of ethnic Vietnamese injection drug users in Melbourne, Australia. *Social Work in Public Health* 24(5), 371–379.

NHS Institute for Innovation and Improvement (2008) *National Library for Health.* Available online: http://www.library.nhs.uk/ [accessed 18 February 2010].

Novakowski, N. & Wellar, B. (2008) Using the Delphi technique in normative planning research: methodological design considerations. *Environment and Planning A* 40, 1485–1500.

O'Brien, A.P., O'Briend, A.J., McNultym N.G., Morrison-Nagatai, E., Skews, G., Ryan, T., Hardy, D.J., Gaskin, C.J. & Boddy, J. (2002) *Clincial Indicators for Mental Health Nursing Standards of Practice in Aotaroal.* New Zealdnnd Report to Health Research Council of New Zealand. Massey University, Palmerston North.

O'Brien, P.W. (1979) *Doctoral Planning Studies: A State of the Art Examination.* Flinders University of South Australia, School of Education Research Seminar, Australia.

Oberst, M. (1978) Priorities in cancer nursing research. *Cancer Nursing* 1, 281–290.

Okamoto, R. (1999) Development of a scale for quality of care management process: a Delphi survey and studies on reliability and validity. *Nippon Koshu Eisei Zasshi / Japanese Journal of Public Health* 46(6), 435–446.

Okoli, C. & Pawlowski, S.D. (2004) The Delphi method as a research tool: an example, design considerations and applications. *Information Management* 42, 15–29.

Ono, R. & Wedemeyer, D.J. (1994) Assessing the validity of the Delphi technique. *Futures* 26(3), 289–304.

Oranga, H.M. & Nordberg, E. (1993) The Delphi panel method for generating health information. *Health Policy and Planning* 8(4), 405–412.

Ota, S., Cron, R., Schanberg, L.E., O'Neil, K., Mellins, E.D., Fuhlbrigge, R.C. & Feldman, B.M. (2008) Research priorities in pediatric rheumatology: The Childhood Arthritis and Rheumatology Research Alliance (CARRA) consensus. *Pediatric Rheumatology* 6(5). Available online: http://www.ped-rheum.com/content/6/1/5 [accessed 15 February 2010].

Owens, C., Ley, A. & Aitken, P. (2008) Do different stakeholder groups share mental health research priorities? A four-arm Delphi study. *Health Expectations* 11(4), 418–431.

Palmer, N. & Batchelor, P. (2006) Informing research in primary dental care: setting priorities. *Primary Dental Care* 13(3) 85–90.

Pallant J. (2007) *SPSS Survival Manual: A Step by Step Guide to Data Analysis Using SPSS*. Open University Press, London.

Parahoo, K. (2006) *Nursing Research: Principals, Processes and Issues* (2nd Edn). Palgrave Macmillan, London.

Parente, F.J. & Anderson-Parente, J.K. (1987) Delphi inquiry systems. In: *Judge Mental Forecasting* (Eds, G. Wright & P. Ayton). John Wiley, Chichester.

Penfield, G. (1975) The relative efficacy of varying applications of face to face interaction versus Delphi in developing consensus about relative priority among goals in student affairs. Unpublished Dissertation, University of Cincinnati. In: *The Delphi Technique: An Experimental Evaluation* (Ed., W. Riggs) (1983). *Technological Forecasting and Social Change* 23, 89–94.

Peters, J., Hutchinson, A., MacKinnon, M., McIntosh, A., Cooke, J. & Jones, R. (2001) What role do nurses play in type 2 diabetes care in the community: a Delphi study. *Journal of Advanced Nursing* 34(2), 179–188.

Pill, J. (1971) The Delphi method: substance, context, a critique and an annotated bibliography. *Socio-Economic Planning Science* 5(1), 57–71.

Pilon, M., Sullivan, S.J. & Coulombe, J. (1995) Persistent vegetative state: which sensory-motor variables should the physiotherapist measure? *Brain Inquiry* 9(4), 365–376.

Pinyeard, B.J., Blair, J.M., Chavez, R. & Stout-Shaffer, S. (1993) Setting a research agenda to promote nursing research. *Clinical Nursing Research* 2(2), 232–239.

Pole, C. & Lampard, R. (2002) *Practical Social Investigation: Qualitative and Quantitative Methods in Social Research*. Prentice Hall, Essex.

Polit, D.F. & Hunger, B.P. (1995) *Nursing Research Principles and Methods*. JB Lippincott Company, Philadelphia.

Polit, D.F. & Hungler, B.P. (1999) *Nursing Research: Principles and Methods*, 6th Edition. Lippincott Company, Philadelphia.

Polit, D., Beck C. & Hungler, B. (2001) *Essentials of Nursing Research – Methods, Appraisal and Utilisation* (5th Edn). JB Lippincott Company, Philadelphia.

Potter, M, Gordon, S. & Hamer, P. (2004) The nominal group technique: a useful consensus methodology in physiotherapy research. *New Zealand Journal of Physiotherapy* 32(3), 126–130.

Powell C. (2003) The Delphi technique: myths and realities. *Journal of Advanced Nursing* 41(4), 376–382.

Preble, J.F. (1983) Public sector use of the Delphi technique. *Technological Forecasting and Social Change* 23(1), 75–88.

Price, B. (2005) Delphi survey research and older people. *Nursing Older People* 17(3), 25–31.

Proctor, S. & Hunt, M. (1994) Using the Delphi survey technique to develop a professional definition of nursing for analysing nursing workload. *Journal of Advanced Nursing* 19, 1003–1014.

Putman, J.W., Spiegel, A.N. & Bruininks, R.H. (1995) Future directions in education and inclusion of students with disabilities: a Delphi investigation. *Exceptional Children* 61(6), 553–576.

Quade, E.S. (1967) *Cost-Effectiveness: Some Trends in Analysis.* Document No P3529. The RAND Corporation, Santa Monica, California.

Raine, S. (2006) Defining the Bobath concept using the Delphi technique. *Physiotherapy Research International* 11(1), 4–13.

Rauch, A., Kirchberger, I., Boldt, C., Cieza, A. & Stucki, G. (2009) Does the Comprehensive International Classification of Functioning, Disability and Health (ICF) Core Set for rheumatoid arthritis capture nursing practice? A Delphi survey. *International Journal of Nursing Studies* 46(10), 1320–1034.

Rauch, W. (1979) The decision Delphi. *Technological Forecasting and Social Change* 15, 159–169.

Reid, N. (1988) The Delphi technique: its contribution to the evaluation of professional practice. In: *Professional Competence and Quality Assurance in the Caring Professions* (Ed., R. Ellis). Croom Helm, London, pp. 230–254.

Rescher, N. (1969) *Delphi and Values.* Document No P4182. The RAND Corporation, Santa Monica, California.

Rescher, R. (1998) *Predicting the Future.* State University of New York Press, Albany, New York.

Richey, J.S., Mar, B.W. & Horner, R. (1985) The Delphi technique in environmental assessment. *Journal of Environmental Management* 21, 135–146.

Rieger, W.G. (1986) Direction in Delphi developments: dissertations and their quality. *Technological Forecasting and Social Change* 29, 195–204.

Riggs, W.E. (1983) The Delphi technique: an experimental evaluation. *Technological Forecasting and Social Change* 23, 89–94.

Rodger, M., Hills, J., Kristjanson, L. & Delphi Study. (2004) A Delphi study on research priorities for emergency nurses in Western Australia. *Journal of Emergency Nursing* 30(2), 117–125.

Rogers, B., Agnew, J. & Pompeii, L. (2000) Occupational health nursing research priorities: a changing focus. *AAOHN, Official Journal of the American association of Occupational Health Nurses* 48(1), 9–16.

Rotondi, A. & Gustafson, D. (1996) Theoretical, methodological and practical issues arising out of the Delphi method. In: *Gazing into the Oracle: the Delphi Method and Its Application to Social Policy and Public Health* (Eds, M. Adler & E. Ziglio). Jessica Kingsley Publishers, Ltd, Bristol, pp. 34–55.

Rowe, G. & Wright, G. (1999) The Delphi technique as forecasting tool: issues and analysis. *International Journal of Forecasting* 15, 353–375.

Rowe, G. & Wright, G. (2001) Expert opinions in forecasting. Role of the Delphi technique. In: *Principles of Forecasting: A Handbook of Researchers and Practitioners* (Ed., J.S. Armstrong). Kluwer Academic Publishers, Boston, pp. 125–144.

Rowe, G., Wright, G. & Bolger, F. (1991) Delphi: a reevaluation of research and theory. *Technological Forecasting and Social Change* 39(3), 235–251.

Rowe, G., Wright, G. & McColl, A. (2005) Judgement change during Delphi-like procedures: the role of majority influence, expertise and confidence. *Technological Forecasting and Social Change* 72, 377–399.

Royal College of Midwives (1995) *Position Paper: The Place of Health Care Assistants in the Maternity Services.* No. 5, October, RCM, London.

Royal College of Midwives (2004) *Prepared to Care: Fit for Purpose Programme.* Preparation of Maternity Care Assistants, RCM Trust, London.

Ruddy, K., Williamson, P., Creed, K. & McNally, M. (1997) *Non Nursing Duties.* I.P.A. Management Development Course. Rotunda Hospital, Dublin.

Rudy, S.F. (1996) A review of Delphi surveys conducted to establish research priorities by speciality nursing organisations from 1985 to 1995. *ORL Head and Neck Nursing* 14(2), 16–24.

Rudy, S.F., Wilkinson, M.A., Dropkin, M.J. & Stevens, G. (1998) Otorhinolaryngology nursing research priorities: results of the 1996/1997 SOHN Delphi survey. *ORL Head, Neck Nursing* 16(1), 14–20.

Sack, J. (1974) *A Test of the Applicability of the Delphi Method of Forecasting As an Aid to Planning in a Commercial Banking Institution.* Unpublished D.B.A. dissertation. Arizona Sate University, Arizona.

Sackman, H. (1974) Delphi assessment: Expert opinion, forecasting, and group process. A report prepared for United States Air Force Project Rand. Rand, Santa Monica, CA.

Sackman, H. (1975) *Delphi-Critique: Expert Opinion, Forecasting and Group Process.* Lexington Books, Massachusetts.

Sadhra, S., Beach, J.R., Aw, T.C. & Sheikh-Ahmed, K. (2001) Occupational health research priorities in Malaysia: a Delphi study. *Occupational and Environmental Medicine* 58(7), 426–431.

Sadleowski, M. (1986) The problem of rigor in qualitative research. *Advanced in Nursing Science* 8(3), 27–37.

Sahal, D. & Yee, K. (1975) Delphi: an investigation from a Bayesian viewpoint. *Technological Forecasting and Social Change* 7, 165–178.

Salmond, S. (1994) Orthopaedic nursing research priorities: a Delphi study. *Orthopaedic Nursing* 13(4), 31–35.

Sandrey, M. & Bulger, S. (2008) The Delphi method: an approach for facilitation evidence based practice in athletic training. *Althetic Training Educación Journal* 3(4), 135–142.

Scheele, D.S. (1975) Reality construction as a product of Delphi interaction. In: *The Delphi Method. Techniques and Applications* (Eds, H.A. Linstone & M. Turoff). Addison-Wesley, London, pp. 37–71.

Scheibe, M. Skutsch, M. & Schofer, J. (1975) Experiments in Delphi methodology. In: *The Delphi Method: Techniques and Applications* (Eds, H.A. Linstone & M. Turoff). Addison-Wesley, Reading, Massachusetts, pp. 257–281.

Schmidt, K., Montgomery, L., Bruene, D. & Kenney, M. (1997) Determining research priorities in pediatric nursing: a Delphi study. *Journal of Pediatric Nursing* 12(4), 201–207.

Schoeman, M.E.F. & Mahajan, V. (1977) Using the Delphi method to assess community health needs. *Technological Forecasting and Social Change* 10(2), 203–210.

Scott, D. & Deadrick, D. (1982) The nominal group technique: applications for training needs assessment. *Training and Development Journal* 26–33.

Scott, E., McMahon, A., Kitson, A. & Rafferty, A.M. (1999) A national initiative to set priorities for R&D in nursing, midwifery and health visiting. Investigating the method. *NT Research* 4(4), 283–290.

Scott, E.A. & Black, N. (1991) When does consensus exist in expert panels? *Journal of Public Health Medicine* 13(1), 36–39.

Sedlak, C., Ross, D., Arslanian, C. & Taggart, H. (1998) Orthopaedic nursing research priorities: a replication and extension. *Orthopaedic Nursing* 17(2), 51–58.

Seyffer, C. (1965) Tomorrow's nurse in a changing world. *International Nursing Review* 12(July/Aug), 66–72.

Sharkey, S.B. & Sharples, A.Y. (2001) An approach to consensus building using the Delphi technique: developing a learning resource in mental health. *Nurse Education Today* 21, 398–408.

Sheikh, A., Major, P. & Holgate, S.T. (2008) Developing consensus on national respiratory research priorities: key findings from the UK Respiratory Research Collaborative e-Delphi exercise. *Respiratory Medicine* 102(8), 1089–1092.

Shepard, J. (1995) Findings of a training needs analysis for qualified nurse practitioners. *Journal of Advanced Nursing* 22, 66–71.

Simoens, S. (2006) Using the Delphi technique in economic evaluation: time to revisit the oracle? *Journal of Clinical Pharmacy and Therapeutics* 31, 519–522.

Sims, L. (1979) Identification and evaluation of competencies of public health nutritionists. *American Journal of Public Health* 69(11), 1099–1105.

Siniscalco, T.M. & Auriat, N. (2005) *Module 8 Questionnaire Design Quanitative Research Methods in Educational Planning*. UNESCO International Instituye for Educacional Planning, France.

Skulmoski, G.J., Hartman, F.T. & Krahn, J. (2007) The Delphi method for graduate research. *Journal of Information Technology Education* 6, 1–21.

Smith, M.W. (1995) Ethics in focus groups: a few concerns. *Qualitative Health Research* 5, 478–486.

Soanes, L, Gibson, F. & Bayliss, J. (2000) Established nursing research priorities on a paediatric haematology, oncology, immunology and infectious diseases unit: a Delphi survey. *European Journal of Oncology Nursing* 4, 108–117.

Soma, M., Hosoi, T. & Yaeda, J. (2009) Exploring high-priority research questions in physical therapy using the Delphi study. *Journal of Physical Therapy Service* 21(4), 367–371.

Sowell, R.L. (2000) Identifying HIV/AIDS research priorities for the next millennium: a Delphi study with nurses in AIDS care. *Journal of the Association of Nursing AIDS Care* 11(3), 42–52.

Spencer-Cooke, B. (1989) Conditions of participation in rural, non-formal education programs: A Delphi study. *Educational Media International*, 26(2), 115–124.

Spivey, B.E. (1971) A technique to determine curriculum content. *Journal of Medical Education* 46, 269–271.

Starkweather, D.B., Gelwicks, L. & Newcomer, R. (1975) Delphi forecasting of health care organization. *Inquiry* 12(1), 37–46.

Stead-Lorenzo, F. (1975) *An Application of the Delphi Method of Forecasting to Nursing Education Planning in West Virginia*. West Virginia University, Michigan.

Steele, R., Bosma, H., Johnston, M.F., Cadell, S., Davies, B., Siden, H. & Straatman, L. (2008) Research priorities in paediatric palliative care: a Delphi study. *Journal of Palliative Care* 24(4), 229–239.

Stetz K.M., Haberman M.R., Holcombe J. & Jones L.S. (1995) 1994 Oncology Nursing Society Research Priorities Survey. *Oncology Nursing Forum* 22, 785–789.

Stevenson, J.S. (1990) Development of nursing knowledge: accelerating the pace. In: *The Nursing Profession Turning Points* (Ed., N.L. Chaska). Mosby, St Louis, pp. 597–606.

Stewart, J. (2001) Is the Delphi technique a qualitative method? *Medicine Education* 35, 922–923.

Stewart, J., O'Halloran, C., Harrigan, P., Spencer, J.A., Barton, J.R. & Singleton, S.J. (1999) Identifying appropriate tasks for the pre-registration year: modified Delphi technique. *British Journal of Medicine* 319(7204), 224–229.

Stewart, T. (1987) The Delphi technique and judgmental forecasting. *Climatic Change* 11, 97–113.

Stez, K., Haberman, M. Holcombe, J., Jones, L. & Moore, K. (1995) 1994 Oncology Nursing Society research Priorities Survey. *Oncology Nursing Forum* 22, 785–789.

Stillwell, J.A. & Hawley, C. (1993) The costs of nursing care. *Journal of Nursing Management* 1(1), 25–50.

Strasser, S., London, L. & Kortenbout, E. (2005) Developing a competence framework and evaluation tool for primary care nurses in South Africa. *Educational Health* 18(2), 133–144.

Strauss, H.J. & Ziegler, L.H. (1975a) The Delphi technique: an adaptive research tool. *British Journal of Occupational Therapy* 61(4), 153–156.

Strauss, H.J. & Ziegler, L.H. (1975b) Delphi, political philosophy and the future. *Futures* 7(3), 184–196.

Streiner, D.L. & Norman, G.R. (1995) Validity. In: *Health measurement Scales: A Practical Guide to Their Development and Use* (Eds, D.L. Streiner & G.R. Norman). Oxford University Press, Oxford, pp. 144–162.

Sullivan, E. & Brye, C. (1983) Nursing's future: use of the Delphi technique for curriculum planning. *Journal of Nurse Education* 22, 187–189.

Sumsion, T. (1998) The Delphi technique: an adaptive research tool. *British Journal of Occupational Therapy* 61(4), 153–156.

Susic, T.P, Svab, I. & Kolsek, M. (2006) Community actions against drinking in Slovenia – a Delphi study. *Drug and Alcohol Dependence* 83, 255–261.

Synnott, G. & McKie, D. (1997) International issues in PR: researching research and prioritizing priorities. *Journal of Public Relations Research* 9(4), 259–282.

Synowiez, B. & Synowiez, P. (1990) Delphi forecasting as a planning tool. *Nursing Management* 21(4), 18–19.

Tapio, P. (2002) Disaggregative policy Delphi: using cluster analysis as a tool for systematic scenario formation. *Technological Forecasting and Social Change* 70, 83–101.

Taylor, R.G., Pease, J. & Reid, W.M. (1990) A study of the survivability and abandonment of contributions in a chain of Delphi rounds. *Psychology: A Study of Human Behaviour* 27, 1–6.

Thangaratinam, S. & Redman, C.W.E. (2005) The Delphi technique. *The Obstetrician and Gynecologist* 7, 120–125.

Thompson, B., MacAuley, D. & McNally, O. (2004) Defining the sports medicine specialist in the United Kingdom: a Delphi study. *British Journal of Sports Medicine* 38, 214–217.

Turoff, M. (1970) The design of a policy Delphi. *Technological Forecasting and Social Change* 2(2), 149–171.

Turoff, M. (1975) The policy Delphi. In: *The Delphi Method. Techniques and Applications* (Eds, H.A. Linstone & M. Turoff). Addison-Wesley, London, pp. 81–101.

Turoff, M. (2006) Personal communication. In: Novakowski, N. & Wellar, B. (2008) Using the Delphi technique in normative planning research: methodological design considerations. *Environment and Planning A* 40, 1485–1500.

Uhl, N.P. (1975) *Consensus and the Delphi Process.* Paper presented at the Annual Meeting of the American Educational Research Association (Washington, DC, April) (ERIC Document ED 104 201).

Ulschak, F.L. (1983) *Human Resource Development: The Theory and Practice of Needs Assessment.* Reston Publishing Company, Inc, Reston, VA.

Van Dijk, M.G.A.J. (1990) Delphi questionnaires versus individual and group interviews: a comparison case. *Technological Forecasting and Social Change* 37, 293–304.

Van Teijlingen, E. & Hundley, V. (2001) *The Importance of Pilot Studies.* Social research UPDATE. Department of Sociology, University of Surrey, Surrey.

van Zolingen, S.J. & Klaassen, C.A. (2003) Selection processes in a Delphi study about key qualifications in senior secondary vocational education. *Technological Forecasting and Social Change* 70, 317–340.

Vazquez-Ramos, R., Leahy, M. & Hernandez N (2009) The Delphi method in rehabilitation counselling research. *Rehabilitation Counseling Bulletin* 50(2), 111–118.

Veal, A.J. (1992) *Research Methods for Leisure and Tourism: a Practical Guide.* Pearson Education, Edinburgh Gate: Harlow, United Kingdom.

Ventura, M.R. & Waligora-Serafin, B. (1981) Study priorities identified by nurses in mental health settings. *International Journal of Nursing Studies* 18(1), 41–46.

Vernon, W. (2009) The Delphi technique: a review. *International Journal of Therapy and Rehabilitation* 16(2), 69–76.

Vogel, I., Brug, J., Van Der Ploeg, C.P.B. & Raat, H. (2009) Prevention of adolescents music induced hearing loss due to discotheque attendance: a Delphi study. *Health Education Research* 24(6), 1043–1050.

Von der Gracht, H.A. (2008) *The Future of LOGISTICS: SCENARIOS for 2025.* Gabler Edition Wissenschaft, Germany.

Walker, A.M. (1994) A Delphi study of research priorities in the clinical practice of physiotherapy. *Physiotherapy* 80(4), 205–207.

Walker, A.M. & Selfe, J. (1996) The Delphi method: a useful took for the allied health researcher. *British Journal of Therapy and Rehabilitation* 3(12), 677–681.

Wang, C.C., Wang, Y., Zhang, K., Fang, J., Liu, W., Luo, S., Tang, S., Wang, S. & Lu, V.C. (2003) Reproductive health indicators for China's rural areas. *Social Science and Medicine* 57(2), 217–225.

Watson, T. (2008) Public relations research priorities: a Delphi study. *Journal of Communication Management* 12(2), 104–123.

Weed, D.L. & McKeown, R.E. (2001) Ethics in epidemiology and public health. *Journal of Epidemiology and Community Health* 55, 855–857.

Weicher, M. (2007) [Name withheld]: Anonymity and its implications. *Proceedings of the American Society for Information Science and Technology* 43(1), 1–11.

Welty, G.A. (1971) *A Critique of the Delphi-Technique.* Proceedings of the American Statistical Association. S. 377–382. Washington D.C.

Welty, G. (1972) Problems of selecting experts for Delphi exercises. *Academy of Management Journal* 15, 121–124.

Whitehead, A.N. (1925) *Science and the Modern World.* McMillan Company, New York.

Whitehead, D. (2005) An international Delphi study examining health promotion and health education in nursing practice, education and policy. *Journal of Clinical Nursing* 17(7), 891–900.

Whitman, N. (1990) The Committee meeting alternative: using the Delphi technique. *Journal of Nurse Administration* 20(pt7/8), 30–36.

Wiegers, T.A. (2006) Adjusting to motherhood. Maternity care assistance during the postpartum period: how to help new mothers cope. *Journal of Neonatal Nursing* 12, 163–171.

Wiener, B., Chacko, S., Brown, T.R., Cron, S.G. & Cohen, M.Z. (2009) Delphi survey of research priorities. *Journal of Nursing Management* 17(5), 532–538.

Wild, C. & Torgersen, H. (2000a) Foresight in medicine: lessons from three European Delphi studies. *European Journal of Public Health* 10(2), 114–119.

Wild, C. & Torgersen, H. (2000b) The Delphi method: a useful too for the allied health researcher. *British Journal of Therapy and Rehabilitation* 3(12), 677–680.

Wilkinson, G. & Williams, P. (1985) Priorities for research on mental health in primary care settings. *Psychological Medicine* 15(3), 507–514.

Williams, P.L. & Webb, C. (1994a) The Delphi Technique: An adaptive research tool. *British Journal of Occupational Therapy* 61(4), 153–156.

Williams, P.L. & Webb, C. (1994b) The Delphi technique: a methodological discussion. *Journal of Advanced Nursing* 19(1), 180–186.

Wilson, A. & Opolski, M. (2009) Identifying barriers to implementing a cardiovascular computerised decision support system (CDSS): a Delphi survey. *Informatics in Primary Care* 17(1), 23–33.

Witkin, B.R. (1984) *Assessing Needs in Educational and Social Programs.* Jossey-Bass Publishers, San Francisco, CA.

Working Group on Priority Setting (2000) Priority setting for health research: lessons from developing countries. *Health Policy and Planning* 15(2), 130–136.

Worthen, B.R. & Saunders, J.R. (1987) *Educational Evaluation: Alternative Approaches and Practical Guidelines.* Longman, New York.

Woudenberg, F. (1991) An evaluation of Delphi. *Technological Forecasting and Social Change* 40, 131–150.

Young, W.H. & Hogben, D. (1978) An experimental study of the Delphi technique. *Education Research Perspective* 5, 57–62.

Yousuf M.I. (2007a) Using experts' opinions through Delphi technique. *Practical Assessment, Research and Evaluation* 12(4). Available online: http://pareonline.net/pdf/v12n4.pdf [accessed 3 February 2009].

Yousuf, M.I. (2007b) The Delphi technique. *Essays in Education* 20, 80–89.

Zeinio, R.N. (1980) Data collection techniques: mail questionnaires. *American Journal of Hospital Pharmacy* 37, 1113–1119.

Ziglio, E. (1996) The Delphi method and its contribution to decision-making. In: *Gazing Into the Oracle: the Delphi Method and Its Application to Social Policy and Public Health* (Eds, M. Alder & E. Ziglio). Jessica Kingsley Publishers, London, pp. 3–33.

Zinn, J., Zalokowski, A. & Hunter, L. (2001) Identifying indicators of laboratory management performance: a multiple consistency approach. *Health Care Management Review* 26, 40–53.

Index

Note: Page numbers with f and t refer to figures and tables respectively.

The Delphi Technique in Nursing and Health Research, First Edition, © S. Keeney,
F. Hasson and H. McKenna   Published 2011 by Blackwell Publishing Ltd.

Printed and bound by CPI Group (UK) Ltd, Croydon, CR0 4YY

27/10/2024

14580396-0002